OXFORD MEDICAL PUBLICATIONS

Paediatric Palliative Medicine

T0177603

Oxford Specialist Handbooks published and forthcoming

Oxford Specialist Handbook of **Paediatric Palliative Medicine**

Second Edition

Richard D.W. Hain

Consultant and Clinical Lead, Paediatric Palliative Care
Noah's Ark Children's Hospital, Cardiff; Visiting Professor,
University of South Wales and Honorary Senior Lecturer,
Bangor University, UK

Satbir Singh Jassal MBE

Medical Director
Rainbows Hospice for Children and Young Adults
Loughborough, UK

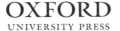

OXFORD
UNIVERSITY PRESS

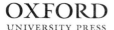

Great Clarendon Street, Oxford, OX2 6DP,
United Kingdom

Oxford University Press is a department of the University of Oxford.
It furthers the University's objective of excellence in research, scholarship,
and education by publishing worldwide. Oxford is a registered trade mark of
Oxford University Press in the UK and in certain other countries

First Edition published 2010
Second Edition published 2016

Impression: 1

Published in the United States of America by Oxford University Press
198 Madison Avenue, New York, NY 10016, United States of America

British Library Cataloguing in Publication Data
Data available

Library of Congress Control Number: 2016934362

ISBN 978–0–19–874545–7

Printed in Great Britain by
Ashford Colour Press Ltd, Gosport, Hampshire

Preface to the Second Edition

It has been more than 5 years since the first edition of the *Oxford Handbook of Paediatric Palliative Medicine*. Reading back over the preface to that edition, it is striking both how much has changed and how much remains the same. The distinctiveness of paediatric palliative care, both from other areas of paediatrics and from our elder sister specialty in adults, is now almost universally acknowledged and now manifests in specialist teams based in hospitals and hospices, not only in the UK but increasingly across the whole world.

It is still true, however, that, for many of those who find themselves having to care for a dying child, it will be a rare event. The aim of this edition of the book, as before, is to equip professionals (and perhaps even some parents) to provide good basic palliative medicine, whether or not they have had formal training or experience with dying children. Its main use will be amongst teams based in hospitals, community paediatric teams, and primary care teams, particularly those who are linked to a children's hospice.

Children's palliative medicine encompasses symptom control but is not limited to it. The book also considers the philosophy and models that support delivery of palliative medicine to children and also the communication and coping skills needed by palliative care professionals. We have revised many of the chapters, rewritten others, and even discarded some. We have added a new chapter on intensive care and significantly expanded the closing formulary section, so that it now includes not only the drugs most used in paediatric palliative care, but also guidelines for using them in symptom control.

As before, if we have succeeded in our aim in writing it, the special usefulness of this handbook in paediatric palliative care, like other specialty handbooks in the OUP series, is a combination of comprehensiveness and portability. Our hope is that it will be an immediate and accessible resource that will help facilitate the practical bedside delivery of effective palliative medicine to children.

Richard D.W. Hain
Satbir Singh Jassal
2016

Contents

Symbols and abbreviations

~	approximately
±	plus or minus
≥	equal to or greater than
≤	equal to or less than
>	greater than
<	less than
≡	equivalent to
%	per cent
®	registered trademark
™	trademark
β	beta
⌘	website
ACE	angiotensin-converting enzyme
ACh	acetylcholine
ACT	Association for Children with Life-threatening or Terminal Conditions and their Families
ADHD	attention-deficit/hyperactivity disorder
AIDS	acquired immune deficiency syndrome
ALT	alanine aminotransferase
APLS	advanced paediatric life support
APPM	Association for Paediatric Palliative Medicine
AST	aspartate aminotransferase
bd	twice daily
BiPAP	bi-level positive airways pressure
BNF	British National Formulary
BNFC	British National Formulary for Children
BP	blood pressure
CaF	Contact a Family
CD	controlled drug
CDOP	Child Death Overview Panel
cf.	compare with
CIVI	continuous intravenous infusion
CNIV	chemotherapy-induced nausea and vomiting
CNS	central nervous system
COX-2	cyclo-oxygenase-2 CH26

CSCI	continuous subcutaneous infusion
CSM	Committee on Safety of Medicines
D_2	dopamine receptor
DEXA	dual-energy X-ray absorptiometry
DMD	Duchenne muscular dystrophy
DNA	deoxyribonucleic acid
DSM-IV	*Diagnostic and Statistical Manual*, fourth edition
EB	epidermolysis bullosa
ECG	electrocardiogram
ECP	emergency care planning
EEG	electroencephalogram
EMA	European Medicines Agency
FBC	full blood count
Fr	French
GAG	glycosaminoglycan
GFR	glomerular filtration rate
GGT	gamma-glutamyl transpeptidase
GORD	gastro-oesophageal reflux disease
GP	general practitioner
h	hour
H^+	hydrogen ion
H1, H2	two types of histamine receptors
HFA	hydrofluoroalkane
HIV	human immunodeficiency virus
HOOF	home oxygen order form CH26
5HT	5-hydroxytryptamine (serotonin; types $5HT_1$, $5HT_2$, etc.)
ICD	International classification of disease
IQ	intelligence quotient
im	intramuscular
INR	international normalized ratio
iv	intravenous
K^+	potassium ion
kcal	kilocalorie
kg	kilogram
L	litre
MAOI	monoamine oxidase inhibitor
MDI	metered dose inhaler
mg	milligram
MHRA	Medicines and Healthcare products Regulatory Agency

min	minute
mL	millilitre
mmol	millimole
MPS	mucopolysaccharide
NaCl	sodium chloride
NB	*nota bene* (take note)
NCA	nurse-controlled analgesia
NCL	neuronal ceroid lipofuscinosis
NG	nasogastric
NHS	National Health Service
NICE	National Institute for Health and Care Excellence
NICU	neonatal intensive care unit
NIPPV	non-invasive positive-pressure ventilation
NMDA	*N*-methyl *D*-aspartate
NSAID	non-steroidal anti-inflammatory drug
od	once daily
OME	oral morphine equivalent
$PaCO_2$	arterial carbon dioxide tension
PCA	patient-controlled analgesia
PDE	principle of double effect
PEG	percutaneous endoscopic gastrostomy
PICU	paediatric intensive care unit
PKU	phenylketonuria
po	orally, by mouth (per os)
PPI	proton pump inhibitor
PPM	paediatric palliative medicine
PONV	post-operative nausea and vomiting
pr	rectally (per rectum)
PRAC	Pharmacovigilance Risk Assessment Committee
prn	*pro re nata* (as required)
PRP	personal resuscitation plan
qds	four times daily
RCPCH	Royal College of Paediatrics and Child Health
s	second
SaO_2	oxygen saturation
sc	subcutaneous
SMA	spinal muscular atrophy
SSRI	selective serotonin re-uptake inhibitor
SVC	superior vena cava

tds	three times daily
U & E	urea and electrolytes
UK	United Kingdom
US	United States
WFI	water for injection
WHO	World Health Organization
w/v	weight by volume

Chapter 1

Paediatric palliative medicine: philosophy and practice

Introduction

This chapter will consider:
- a brief history of palliative care in children;
- a definition of palliative care in children;
- how that might need to be worked out in the practical care of children with life-limiting conditions.

History

The history of the development of children's palliative care has been a slow evolution over the last 35 years. Since the Second World War, medicine has advanced so much and so fast that there seems to be optimism that anything could be healed. This has led many doctors to have difficulties when dealing with children and families where life is limited and treatments are by definition unsuccessful. In the years before the development of the palliative care movement, a lot of good work was already done by community and hospital paediatricians, often with limited resources. The convergence of a number of different threads has acted as a catalyst to the development of paediatric palliative care:

- the recognition of the need for, and development of, adult palliative care;
- the development of multidisciplinary care at home and in the community by paediatric oncology, and later other paediatric subspecialties;
- the opening of the first children's hospice Helen House in 1982 in Oxford UK;
- changing attitudes amongst doctors and nurses towards communication with children and families, in particular recognizing that their wishes on the type and location of care are important;
- an understanding of the importance of teamworking at health level, but also at social and educational levels.

Paediatric palliative care is now an emerging subspecialty within medical care of children. There are children's hospices throughout the world. In these and other parts of the world, paediatric palliative care is also being provided in hospitals and in the community by paediatricians, family doctors, and adult palliative care doctors. The models of care used are based on the local needs and resources.[1]

The number of child deaths is disproportionately high in resource-poor countries. It is vital that we all recognize the need to support the teams providing palliative care to children in these under-resourced areas of the world. As such, we have endeavoured to incorporate advice for these parts of the world in this handbook.

Children are not just small adults. When we manage children, we have to understand issues such as:

- differing physiology and pharmacodynamics;
- ethical issues around autonomy and consent;
- changes associated with development and growth;
- family dynamics;
- differing medical conditions, timescales, and symptom presentation;
- intensity of grief and bereavement;
- the limited numbers of life-limited children in developed countries, and hence limited experience of the health-care professionals.

Definition

The Royal College of Paediatrics and Child Health (RCPCH) and the Association for Children with Life-threatening or Terminal Conditions and their Families (ACT, now Together for Short Lives) define palliative care as:

- ' ... an active and total approach to the care of children, embracing physical, emotional, social and spiritual elements'.[2,3]

So palliative care is:

- active (it is not simply a cessation of treatment); and
- total (it seeks to address the child's whole experience of symptoms, rather than dividing them arbitrarily into physical, emotional, spiritual symptoms).

The American Academy of Pediatrics definition states that paediatric palliative care:

- ' ... includes the control of pain and other symptoms and addresses the psychological, social or spiritual problems of children and their families'.[4]

While this is similar to the ACT/RCPCH definition, it is perhaps less satisfactory, as it suggests that symptom control is a mainly physical phenomenon, somehow separate from psychological, social, and spiritual problems.

Practical applications

A major dilemma facing paediatric palliative care in the UK currently is identifying which children we should be caring for. This dilemma arises from the following issues.

- Medical intervention often leads to children living longer, e.g. up to 40 years of age with cystic fibrosis and up to 24 years of age with ventilation in Duchenne muscular dystrophy (DMD).
- Many children may have severe static neurological problems and not be expected to die in childhood but would still need or benefit from palliative care.
- Predicting life expectancy is notoriously difficult and unreliable in paediatrics.
- A number of neurodegenerative or genetic disorders cannot be identified so, without a label of diagnosis, prognosis becomes unpredictable.

How should the basic principles be put into practice in order to address these issues practically?

From the basic definition, three practical principles can be derived that need to underlie paediatric palliative medicine (PPM) practice.

- Need to balance harm and benefit. All interventions in children with life-limiting conditions should plausibly do them more good than harm.
- A rational approach is a compassionate one. The principles of good medicine are as important in caring for dying children as in paediatrics generally. A rational approach is the way to ensure the best benefit for the least side effects.
- Palliative medicine is 'holistic'. Palliative care needs to address all the dimensions of a child's experience, not just the physical.
- Combining these three principles means that sometimes good palliative medicine will mean balancing physical benefits against (for example) spiritual ones.

Balance of harm and benefit

For any intervention contemplated:
- there will be a negative impact of some kind or kinds;
- there will also be beneficial effects;
- the first responsibility of the palliative medicine physician is to consider whether the harm to the patient outweighs the benefit;
- it may mean balancing benefits and harms of different kinds (for example, weighing physical benefit against emotional harm).

Example: In addressing the possible place of palliative chemotherapy, the potential benefits are:
- the existential value of 'doing something';
- the possibility of prolonging the valuable life;
- the possibility of relieving pain.

Adverse effects are:
- physical effects of neutropenia;
- need for admission, hair loss, and feeling unwell;
- need for frequent attendances at hospital for drugs and/or blood tests;
- loss of normality.

In considering whether palliative chemotherapy is justified, palliative medicine physicians need to look at physical, psychosocial, and spiritual issues on both sides of the balance.

This is complicated further.
- The World Health Organization (WHO) approach provides pain relief for most patients without the need for palliative chemotherapy.
- For some families, the process of prolonging life will be, or will be seen as, a process of prolonging death. Not only is prolonging life not a benefit, it may actually be seen as a positive harm.

Decision-making in PPM demands careful and thoughtful consideration of the needs of the individual patient, remembering as far as possible to encompass all dimensions of his or her individual experience. The corollary is that there is no such thing as an intervention that is always inappropriate. It will depend on the individual child's individual experiences at a specific time.

Commencing morphine is sometimes, quite wrongly, considered an automatic response to acknowledgement that treatment is palliative. In reality, the same careful balance needs to be considered.
- Harms:
  - physical (e.g. constipation);
  - psychosocial (e.g. medicalization);
  - existential/spiritual (e.g. the assumption that morphine implies impending death).
- Benefits:
  - physical (e.g. relief of physical pain);
  - psychosocial (e.g. relief from dyspnoea);
  - existential/spiritual (e.g. effects of better sleep).

A rational approach: reforming the 'medical model'

A rational approach is always logical.

An example is the need to make a diagnosis of pain before treating it. The WHO pain ladder is the gold standard for managing pain in palliative care. It depends critically on prescribing an appropriate adjuvant at each stage of the ladder. There is a good evidence basis for use of adjuvants, *providing they are used for the appropriate pain syndrome*. It is therefore important to distinguish between pain syndromes on the basis of history and examination findings.

- A rational approach is always evidence-based, where possible. Where there is evidence, clearly we must be guided by it if we are to do the best for our patients.
- However, it would not be rational only to do things for which we have a substantial evidence base. The rational response, in the absence of evidence, is to do what is logical and has worked before.

Evidence-based palliative medicine

The evidence basis in palliative medicine is generally weak, and especially so in the paediatric specialty.[5] Clinical practice in PPM is underpinned by three levels of evidence.

Good evidence

See the Cochrane database. There are relatively few examples, e.g.:
- use of oral morphine;
- the WHO pain ladder;
- anticonvulsants and antidepressants as adjuvants in neuropathic pain.

Evidence extrapolated from other contexts

Extrapolation is often from other paediatric specialties such as management of acute pain, or chemotherapy-related nausea and vomiting.

Example: patient-controlled analgesia (PCA)
- Little published evidence in palliative care; BUT
- Overwhelming evidence of usefulness in acute pain.

PCA is a logical and rational treatment, either as a way of delivering the WHO approach or as a second line if that approach fails.

Little clinical evidence but plausible

Sometimes it is necessary to proceed, not on the basis of evidence, but on the basis that, with a sound understanding of symptom pathophysiology and therapeutics, effectiveness is plausible.

Example: neuropathic adjuvants in bone pain
The effectiveness of neuropathic agents for bone pain in paediatric palliative care is unproven, but rational because:
- certain adjuvants (including ketamine and gabapentin) are known to be effective in neuropathic pain because of an effect on nerve stimulation;
- it is known that distortion of the microarchitecture of bone results in stimulation of pain receptors;

- it is logical that neuropathic adjuvants may also be effective as an adjuvant in bone pain;
- this is borne out in some laboratory studies;

So a rational approach would dictate that, while they should not be considered as first-line treatment in bone pain, anti-neuropathic pain agents should be tried if first-line approaches fail.[6] Furthermore, clinical trials should be designed to demonstrate the possibility of a wider use.

A general approach

More generally, to construct a logical and rational approach (rather than a strictly evidence-based one), we should:
- start with what we know works (e.g. the WHO guidelines);
- if that fails, use a logical extrapolation from evidence in related areas (e.g. PCA in acute pain);
- if that fails, be creative, based on a sound understanding of pharmacology and therapeutics and of laboratory studies (e.g. anti-neuropathic agents in bone pain);
- continually generate well-designed clinical research questions, and trials to answer them.

But:
- we do not have carte blanche to use any drug in any way we choose;
- we should always be sceptical of new approaches. It would not serve the interests of our patients if we took at face value the conclusions of a few case studies or a visit from a drug rep. Palliative care is particularly vulnerable to the seduction of new approaches, because we deal with such a range of symptoms with such a weak evidence base;
- it would be equally wrong to discount new approaches completely. Some will become the standard approach of the future. Fentanyl patches, now the standard second-line approach in palliative care pain, were once novel and untried.

WHO pain ladder
- The WHO pain ladder is the gold standard approach to the pain of palliative care in children.
- Although it first appeared in the 1998 publication *Cancer pain relief and palliative care in children*,[7] little in it is specific to cancer pain.
- As pain intensity increases, so simple analgesics should give way to simple analgesics with low-dose opioids, and, once these doses no longer control the pain, low-dose opioids should be replaced with opioids at higher dose.
- At each stage of the ladder, an appropriate adjuvant should be introduced. They should not be delayed until opioids have failed.

Multidimensionality ('holism')

The third basic principle is that palliative medicine should address all dimensions of a patient's experience. In paediatric palliative care, management of symptoms may be easy. Providing high-quality care, on the other hand, is very difficult. It requires doctors to break out of the traditional pathophysiological paradigm and look at a more holistic problem-solving framework.

Dictionary definitions suggest that holism is: 'the view that a whole system of beliefs must be analysed rather than simply its individual components' and 'the theory of the importance of taking all of somebody's physical, mental, and social conditions into account in the treatment of illness'.

Multidimensionality does *not* mean categorizing each symptom as 'physical', 'spiritual', or 'psychosocial'. Rather, it means recognizing that all experiences, including symptoms, exist simultaneously in all three dimensions, which must therefore be considered.

- Physical aspects of an experience can be characterized by the questions 'what is happening to me?' and 'what can be done to stop it?'.
- Psychosocial aspects can be characterized by the questions 'how will this affect my life?' and 'how do I feel about that?'.
- Existential (or spiritual) questions can be characterized by the questions 'why is this happening to me?' and 'what does it mean?'.

In practical terms, a multidimensional or holistic approach means:
- looking at the child, his or her family, and the world around them to determine care;
- looking beyond the physical, at the emotional, spiritual, and environmental;
- accepting that many different professionals may have skills and experience that would benefit the child and to value this diversity of support (Fig. 1.1);
- appreciating the expertise that parents have in looking after their child;
- valuing the support grandparents, family, friends, school, church, and faith can give to the child.

Teamworking is not easy but is attainable with effort (see ➲ Chapters 22 and 23).

Faced with the reality of a dying child ...
- Do not panic; do not dive in blindly; keep your hands tucked behind your back, your mouth shut, and listen to the parents. While no one can always know for sure, the parents are the people most likely to know what their child is experiencing.
- Only once you have obtained a good history from all sources should you start an examination. Be methodical, logical, and, above all, professional—the parents have allowed you into their lives, because they perceive that you may be able to help them. A careful examination is part of what they expect, and are reassured by, in a doctor.
- Once you have formulated a plan of action, go through it with the parents in a language that they understand, offering a range of alternatives where appropriate. Parents' sense that they have an

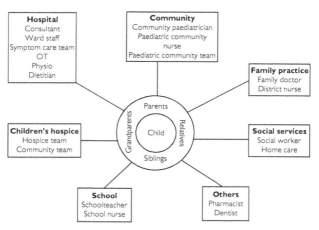

Fig. 1.1 Professional involvement in the care of a child.

informed choice in the care of their dying child is supportive both before and after the child's death.

• The preferences of parents are extremely important, but they are not determinative. Usually the interests of parents and child are the same, but not always. The right approach is the one that best serves the child's interests.

• Document and disseminate information to all your care team. Check that they are happy about the care plan and that everyone is clear about their role.

Summary of paediatric palliative medicine

Palliative care in children is:
- active—not just a cessation of curative treatment, but the active introduction of other approaches;
- total—recognizing all dimensions of all experience, particularly symptoms.

There are three underlying principles that should always inform management:
- the need to balance harm and benefit (sometimes need to balance physical benefits against psychosocial or spiritual harms);
- the need for a rational approach (always logical, evidence-based, where possible, but empirical where necessary);
- the need for a multidimensional approach, remembering that all experiences occupy all dimensions.

References

1. Knapp, C., Woodworth, L., Wright. M., Downing. J., Drake, R., Fowler-Kerry, S., et al. (2011). Pediatric palliative care provision around the world: a systematic review. Pediatr. Blood Cancer 57 (3), 361–8.
2. Association for Children with Life-threatening or Terminal Conditions and their Families (ACT) and Royal College of Paediatrics and Child Health (RCPCH) (1997). A guide to the development of children's palliative care services, first edition. ACT and RCPCH, Bristol and London.
3. Association for Children with Life-threatening or Terminal Conditions and their Families (ACT) and Royal College of Paediatrics and Child Health (RCPCH) (2003). A guide to the development of children's palliative care services—updated report, second edition. ACT and RCPCH, Bristol and London.
4. Committee on Bioethics and Committee on Hospital Care (2000). Palliative care for children. Pediatrics 106 (2), 351–7.
5. Colvin, L. and Fallon, M. (2008). Challenges in cancer pain management—bone pain. Eur. J. Cancer 44 (8), 1083–90.
6. Beecham, E., Candy, B., Howard, R., McCulloch, R., Laddie, J., Rees, H., et al. (2015). Pharmacological interventions for pain in children and adolescents with life-limiting conditions. Cochrane Database Syst. Rev. 3, CD010750.
7. World Health Organization, in collaboration with the International Association for the Study of Pain (1998). Guidelines for analgesic drug therapy. In: Cancer pain relief and palliative care in children, pp. 24–8. World Health Organization, Geneva.

Chapter 2

Models of paediatric palliative care

Introduction

The United Kingdom (UK) has a variety of resources for children with life-limiting conditions that are perhaps unrivalled in the world. This is both good and bad. It offers the potential for children and their families to have choices about the location of their care. On the other hand, a multiplicity of agencies brings with it the risk of miscommunication and internecine strife.

The ideal model for providing palliative care to children with life-limiting conditions would offer:

- a choice of location;
- a range of care skills, encompassing health care and non-health care, professional and volunteer, and specialist and generalist;
- an environment in which it is possible to address a child's and family's needs in an unhurried and thorough manner;
- access to medical expertise that includes excellent primary care, as well as specialist palliative care, for children;
- care that is free at the point of need;
- care that is available to all children with life-limiting conditions.

It is probably impossible for any single agency to provide all these alone. The model is, in practice, one of cooperation between many different agencies. For this to function effectively requires mutual respect for the services each can provide and, above all, good and sensitive inter-professional communication.

Who needs it?

The early definition of palliative medicine sprang from adults and focused largely on cancer. The range of life-limiting conditions in childhood is much broader than in the adult specialty and does not focus on malignant conditions.

RCPCH/ACT categories

In 1997, the RCPCH, together with ACT, addressed this misconception by defining four categories of life-limiting conditions in childhood which:
- broaden the understanding of the need for access to palliative care services by including:
  - some children for whom cure is possible but not certain;
  - some children who are currently well but will inevitably deteriorate.
  - some children whose underlying condition is not progressive but will nevertheless cause premature death.
- form the basis for clinical service development and research in the UK;
- are flexible enough to accommodate any life-limiting condition;
- are difficult to validate, since the categories describe disease trajectories, rather than comprising lists of specific conditions. The RCPCH/ACT categories form the basis for a Directory of life-limiting conditions.

Category I

Includes children whose condition may be curable, but, at diagnosis, the possibility of death is significant.
- Examples are cancer and congenital heart disease.
- Of all categories, most closely resembles adult palliative medicine.
- Accounts for approximately one-third of children needing active palliative care at any one time.

Category II

Includes children whose disease will certainly kill them prematurely, but only after a period of normality during which they may need no palliative care at all.
- Examples include DMD and cystic fibrosis.
- Accounts for approximately one-sixth of children needing active palliative care at any one time.

Category III

Describes children with conditions whose course is relentlessly progressive from the moment diagnosis is made, if not before.
- Includes metabolic conditions such as mucopolysaccharidosis, Batten's disease, and juvenile Huntington's disease.
- Accounts for approximately one-sixth of children needing active palliative care at any one time.

Category IV

Includes children with conditions that are not themselves progressive, but with effects that are cumulative over time and will inevitably restrict the child's lifespan.
- Includes cerebral palsy and severe epilepsy.

- The child will typically experience four or five acute 'end of life' episodes.
- Extraordinarily heterogeneous group, perhaps least like adult palliative care.
- Characterized by extreme unpredictability and numerous 'rehearsals' for a terminal phase before death actually occurs.
- Accounts for at least one-third of children with life-limiting conditions.

Epidemiology

- Using the RCPCH/ACT definitions, the prevalence of life-limiting conditions in children in England is 32 per 10 000.
- That equates to ~40 000 children in England with life-limiting conditions who need access to palliative care services.
- That number increased by 23% between 2000 and 2010, and is likely to continue to increase as a result of medical technology.
- Around half of all deaths in childhood occur from life-limiting conditions.
- The prevalence of life-limiting conditions is higher where there is social deprivation and in non-white UK populations.

Children's hospices

Children's hospices offer a unique and greatly valued resource to children with life-limiting conditions. The UK has around 50 children's hospices. Their services are usually provided at no cost either to the patient or to the Trust. It is very important that paediatricians support hospices and work with them, if seamless palliative care for children is to be achieved.

- Identified by most families as an invaluable resource.
- Typically custom-built facilities, providing excellent environment for multidimensional care.
- Typically house 5–15 children.
- High staff-to-patient ratio.
- Combines many benefits of a hospital, but in a much more 'home-like' environment.
- Main emphasis is on specialist respite.
- Medical needs of children in hospice range from primary care to specialist paediatric palliative medicine. Ideally, therefore, medical support should be available from both general practitioners (GPs) and paediatricians.
- Many GPs in children's hospices have undertaken postgraduate training in PPM.
- Increasingly, hospices offer specialist PPM through arrangements with the local tertiary PPM team.
- Typically little statutory funding, so operate independently of Trusts (this independence can be valued by families).
- Provide a wide range of services, often including complementary therapies.
- Most provide these only for their own patients.

Paediatric palliative medicine specialists

- Have completed subspecialty training in PPM (APPM level 4).
- Currently fewer than 20 consultants in PPM in the UK.
- Most based in tertiary paediatric centres in major cities.
- Liaise with all providers of palliative care to children whenever specialist palliative medicine is required (Fig. 2.1).
- See patients at home, hospital, hospice, and school, and in outpatients.

Paediatrician or general practitioner with special interest in palliative medicine

- Currently around 100 in the UK.
- Usually has workload in related discipline, especially primary care, community paediatrics, paediatric oncology, neurodisability, or neurology.
- Has completed appropriate postgraduate training (APPM level 3).
- May have completed formal special interest ('SPIN') training.

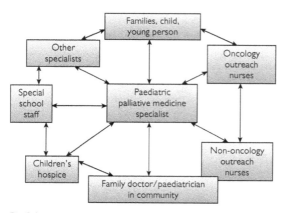

Fig. 2.1 Role of the PPM specialist is to work with, and to support, all agencies providing palliative care for children in all environments in which the child finds herself.

Summary of models of paediatric palliative care

An ideal model of palliative care would allow:
- expert care to follow the child, wherever the child is;
- good access to specialist medical and nursing expertise in palliative care;
- choice for family and child of inpatient- or outpatient-based management.

This requires a model that is either:
- community-based, reaching into the hospital;
- hospital- or hospice-based, reaching out to the home and school; or
- a combination of the two.

Given the variety of models that have developed, the last of these is the most common prevailing approach in the UK.

Further reading

Association for Children with Life-threatening or Terminal Conditions and their Families (ACT) and Royal College of Paediatrics and Child Health (RCPCH) (1997). *A guide to the development of children's palliative care services*, first edition. ACT and RCPCH, Bristol and London.

Baba, M. and Hain, R. (2012). Paediatric palliative care in the United Kingdom. In: Knapp, C., Madden, V., and Fowler-Kerry, S., editors. *Pediatric palliative care: global perspectives*, pp. 269–98. Springer, Amsterdam.

Fraser, L.K., Miller, M., Hain, R., Norman, P., Aldridge, J., McKinney, P.A., et al. (2012). Rising national prevalence of life-limiting conditions in children in England. *Pediatrics* **129** (4), e923–9.

Hain, R., Devins, M., Hastings, R., and Noyes, J. (2013). Paediatric palliative care: development and pilot study of a 'Directory' of life-limiting conditions. *BMC Palliat. Care.* **12** (1), 43.

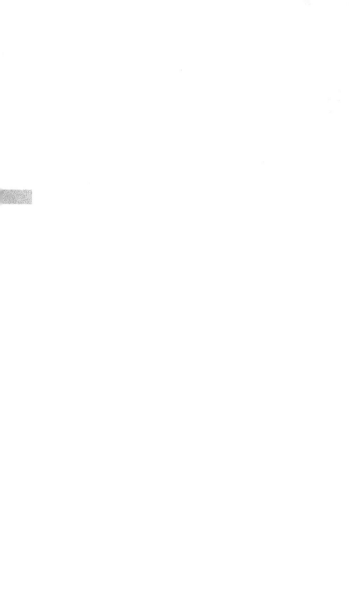

Ethics in palliative care

Introduction

Ethics does not provide a rigid 'machine' for the resolution of complex decisions, into which a difficult clinical question can be fed into one end and a correct answer extracted from the other. Nor should the palliative phase be seen as a time when ordinary ethical principles no longer apply and when anything is permissible, providing the intention is good.

Ethical principles are the same in palliative medicine as they are in other medical disciplines. Clinical decisions at the end of life, however, may involve ethical considerations and judgements that are particularly complex and on whose outcome much may depend.

Review of basic ethical principles

Principlism

Four basic medical ethical principles were articulated by Beauchamp and Childress. The principles are not fundamental ethical 'laws', analogous to the laws of pharmacology. Rather, they are useful practical summaries of more complex underlying ideas, analogous to a formulary. They are:
1. beneficence (an obligation for doctors to do good for their patients);
2. non-maleficence (an obligation for doctors to avoid doing harm to their patients);
3. respect for autonomy (an obligation for doctors to ensure a patient feels valued and respected as an individual);
4. justice as fairness (an obligation for doctors to give equal value to their patients).

There is no hierarchy of principles; all are equally important. To these can usefully be added a fifth:[1]
5. Attention to scope (the obligation to consider the application of these principles to the individual, patient-specific situation).

Palliative medicine

The underlying principles of palliative medicine (see → Chapter 1) are:
- the need to balance burden and benefit;
- the need for a rational approach;
- the need for multidimensionality (holism).

It follows that:
- since all palliative interventions carry the possibility of both good and bad effects, the principles of beneficence and non-maleficence require that a judgement be made about the relative risk;
- a rational judgement requires that interventions should be carried out if the potential benefit probably outweighs the potential burden;
- the extent and limitations of evidence in respect of these must be known; the existing evidence base should be accessed by clinicians and utilized in a rational manner;
- both benefits and burdens need to be considered in all dimensions (physical, spiritual, and psychosocial);
- in the absence of possibility of cure, benefits in one dimension might need to be balanced against burdens in another. For some patients, on some occasions, this may mean prioritizing quality of life over its duration, or even over the chance for cure;
- since such judgements involve subjective experience, it is necessary to canvass and give weight to the views of the child and family in making them;
- service delivery systems may need to be modified to allow equal access by all those who could benefit;
- decision-making should be honest, transparent, justifiable, and well recorded.

Principle of double effect

Double effect is an important principle in palliative care.[2]
- The principle of double effect is that an act is permissible, even if the outcome is undesirable and known beforehand to be possible, *providing*:
  - the intended act is good;
  - the bad outcome was not the main intention;
  - the good effect is a direct consequence of the action, rather than an incidental consequence of the bad effect;
  - the good effect must be sufficiently desirable to outweigh the bad one.
- The principle of double effect (PDE) recognizes that all interventions have both good and bad effects, and that it is not possible to know with certainty beforehand which will occur.
- It was famously articulated by the Catholic moral theologian Thomas Aquinas in the thirteenth century, but it is a matter of observation and derivable from first principles—there is no casuistry involved.

It therefore follows that:
- the PDE does not equate with, or of itself permit, euthanasia;
- most prescribing of medications in any context illustrates double effect, since there is always the small possibility of an unintended and adverse reaction occurring, for which the prescriber is not morally culpable;
- the PDE is particularly important at the end of life, both because prolongation of life may not be a priority and improvement in life quality assumes a greater importance.

Public perception is sometimes, quite wrongly, that PDE means doctors can, and do, hasten death through palliative medications. While it has traditionally been uncommon for those working in palliative care to have to justify their clinical decisions and actions in court, this is beginning to change. Fear of litigation should not lead clinicians to become overcautious, but it is important to ensure that:
- documentation is always clear, dated, and signed;
- drug doses are appropriate for the severity of the symptom;
- drug doses given are recorded, irrespective of who administers them;
- hospital and primary care records are kept up-to-date, irrespective of where the child is cared for;
- there is early involvement (if necessary through telephone support) of appropriate professional skills that will usually include specialist paediatrics and palliative medicine, as well as primary care;
- any departure from established palliative medicine practice (i.e. the WHO approach; see ⊃ Chapter 4) is documented and justified, especially with respect to opioid initiation, titration, and maintenance.

Withholding and withdrawing treatment

If:

- 'doing good' means more than simply finding a cure; and
- 'doing harm' is an inevitable part of some treatments,

then it follows that, in palliative care, sometimes balancing burden and bene-fit, it is in a child's interest to withhold or withdraw medical treatments, even where they might prolong life. That might include artificial nutrition, ventilation, or hydration.

The circumstances under which that might occur are explored in the RCPCH 2015 publication *Making decisions to limit treatment in life-limiting and life-threatening conditions in children: a framework for practice.*

- Rigid rules, even for conditions that seem hopeless, should be avoided. The RCPCH document (2015):

  ' ... sets out circumstances under which withholding or withdrawing life-sustaining treatment might be ethically permissible - NOT circumstances under which such treatment *must* certainly be withheld or withdrawn. In particular it describes situations in which individual children should be spared inappropriate invasive procedures - NOT *types* of children to whom *appropriate* procedures should be denied.'

- Ultimately, the key consideration is always what is in the child's interests. There is probably a morally relevant difference between 'interests' and 'best interests', but no intervention is justified if it will cause the child more harm than good, even if it is requested by the child's parents.
- Decisions should never be rushed and should be made by the whole team, in discussion with families and with all available evidence. Where there is a clinical ethics committee, their opinion should be sought at the earliest opportunity.
- Any decision to withhold or withdraw curative therapy should be accompanied by consideration of the child's palliative or end-of-life care needs.
- In emergencies, it is often doctors in training who are called on to resuscitate. Unless there is clearly documented evidence that forward planning discussions (such as advance or emergency care plans) have taken place, life-sustaining treatment should usually be administered and continued until a senior and more experienced doctor arrives.

The legal status of advice given by clinical ethics committees and other pro-fessional bodies, such as Royal Colleges, is largely established by case law and is therefore subject to change. Nevertheless, demonstration of good professional practice will always lend weight to clinical decisions, however ethically challenging. Such good practice includes:

- consistent and clear documentation;
- evidence that the child's and/or family's views have been canvassed and given weight;
- evidence of discussion with colleagues on the health-care team;
- reference to published guidelines;
- evidence of discussion with the clinical ethics committee;
- evidence of careful consideration of burden and benefit in all dimensions;
- above all, consistent evidence that the child's own best interests have been made paramount.

Euthanasia

Euthanasia has come to refer to the active hastening of death through medical intervention. It is illegal in children in most countries but is permitted in Holland and Belgium. Governments elsewhere, including in the UK, are under pressure to review the law to permit euthanasia. Broadly speaking, its adherents make three arguments:

- *compassion (beneficence)*: the life of a child is so unpleasant for them that death is in her interests and should be offered;
- *autonomy*: if the parents of a child with a life-limiting condition do not want to care for her, they should be allowed that choice;
- *justice*: the care of children with life-limiting conditions is expensive in a way that is out of proportion to the contribution they will make to society.

A fourth, more minoritarian, claim is that euthanasia is already practised and so should be regulated. The nature of the claim means there can be no evidence to support it.

Although each of the arguments has some merit, they are all based on particular beliefs and ideologies, namely:

- that it is possible to know a child's experience of their own life in some measurable way;
- that the authority of parents to speak for their child derives from their 'ownership' of the child—that is, the child's interests are those of the parents;
- that the primary purpose of health care is to maximize the contribution individuals can make to society.

Those beliefs and ideologies are problematic because:

- there is no clear relationship between what can be observed about a child and how much she enjoys her life. Severely disabled children who can do so often report a good quality of life. Furthermore, it is extremely rare for any patient's suffering to remain intractable in the face of adequate access to good palliative care;
- parents have no moral authority to request interventions that will harm their child. Parental 'authority' is logically limited to:
  - giving advice as to what interventions are appropriate, on the basis of their expert knowledge of the child;
  - giving permission for interventions that will be in their child's interest.
- the primary purpose of health care is to restore an individual to health, considered broadly as the best quality of life it is possible for her to have within the constraints of her condition.

There are also important dangers in giving some people the legal authority to take the life of others.

- It is hard to legislate safely, because legislation relies on terms that are unclear, either because they lack objectively true meaning (such as the claim that someone has 'unbearable suffering') or else are meaningless in practice (such as the shamanic pronouncement that someone is 'within 6 months of death').

- It represents a prejudice against disabled people, rather than just against disability, because the law would codify a different acceptable threshold for taking the life of one person from another, solely on the basis of her condition.
- It represents an exploitation of the vulnerable, because health-care resources saved by taking the life of children with life-limiting conditions would be used for the benefit of patients who were already stronger and healthier.
- It provides opportunities for individuals to coerce others into requesting that a life be ended, either deliberately or inadvertently (for example, by expressing exhaustion after a bad night's sleep).
- There is no protection against cultural coercion—that is, the pressure to conform that is exerted on an individual by society (for example, if it were seen as normal for parents to euthanize children with Edwards, it would be more difficult for a parent to choose instead to care for their particular child).

It is important to recognize that most adherents of euthanasia are motivated by compassion. Considered rationally, however, euthanasia is an extremely bad idea.

Summary of ethics in palliative care

- Beauchamp and Childress' Four Principles are currently the basis of medical ethics. They are neither a solution machine nor a consistent moral theory, but represent complex underlying philosophical arguments and need to be specified for the individual context.
- The PDE is important in end-of-life care, because it acknowledges the importance of intention (shaped by competence), as well as outcome. In symptom control, the PDE relies on the use of proportionate doses of rationally selected medications.
- All interventions carry harm. For some interventions, under some circumstances, that harm outweighs the benefit. Such an intervention is against the child's interests and should be withheld or withdrawn. More often, the balance is not clear, and withholding or withdrawing the intervention is reasonable but not mandatory.
- Euthanasia is the legalized killing of one person by another. It is currently illegal in most countries. Proponents of a change that would legalize euthanasia are usually motivated by compassion, and their arguments invoke the principles of beneficence, autonomy, or justice. Because they often flow from specific, more fundamental, ideological conceptions, however, many of the arguments are deeply problematic. In the view of the authors, euthanasia is both unnecessary and dangerous.

References

1. Gillon, R. (1994). Medical ethics: four principles plus attention to scope. *Br. Med. J.* **309** (6948), 184–8.
2. Fohr, S.A. (1998). The double effect of pain medication: separating myth from reality. *J. Palliat. Med.* **1** (4), 315–28.

Further reading

Beauchamp, T. and Childress, J. (2009). *Principles of biomedical ethics*, sixth edition. Oxford University Press, New York.
Hain, R.D. (2014). Euthanasia: 10 myths. *Arch. Dis. Child.* **99** (9), 798–9.
Larcher, V., Craig, F., Bhogal, K., Wilkinson, D., Brierley, J.; Royal College of Paediatrics and Child Health (2015). Making decisions to limit treatment in life-limiting and life-threatening conditions in children: a framework for practice. *Arch. Dis. Child.* **100** Suppl 2, s3–23.
Verhagen, E. and Sauer, P.J. (2005). The Groningen protocol—euthanasia in severely ill newborns. *N. Engl. J. Med.* **352** (10), 959–62.

Pain: introduction

Introduction

Definition
- Pain is: 'an unpleasant sensory and emotional experience associated with actual or potential tissue damage, or described in terms of such damage'.[1]
- A more succinct definition that similarly emphasizes pain's subjective nature is 'pain is whatever the patient says it is'.[2]

The key points in any definition of pain are as follows.
- It is subjective and cannot be properly diagnosed or evaluated using any objective means.
- It is usually interpreted as being the result of tissue damage.
- It is not, in reality, necessarily associated with tissue damage.
- It occurs independently of the child's capacity to express it.

Classification
There are many systems for classifying pain. They may be based on:
- duration of pain (acute versus chronic);
- intensity (severe, moderate, mild);
- presumed pathophysiology (visceral, somatic, sympathetic mediated);
- location (headache, stomach ache, backache, etc.);
- sensitivity to opioids.

In palliative medicine, the most widely used classification is pragmatic, based on recognizable clusters of pain symptoms that are associated with response to specific therapeutic interventions:
- neuropathic: characterized by disordered sensation, responsive to adjuvants such as anticonvulsants and antidepressants;
- bone pain: characterized by intense and focal nature, responsive to adjuvants such as non-steroidal anti-inflammatory drugs (NSAIDs) and bisphosphonates;
- muscle spasm: characterized by responsiveness to muscle relaxants and antispasmodics;
- cerebral irritation: characterized by association with acute brain injury and signs of anxiety, responsive to adjuvants such as benzodiazepines.

Pain is also sometimes considered according to how sensitive it is to opioids:
- opioid-sensitive;
- opioid-insensitive (or resistant);
- opioid-partially resistant.

Total pain
Total pain describes the concept that pain, of any physical origin or none, occurs in the broader context of an individual's life at that moment.
This means it is influenced by:
- the severity of any physical tissue damage;
- its impact on function and how the child and/or family feels about it (psychosocial and emotional);
- what pain means to them and any explanations they construct for it (spiritual, or existential).

Attention to one dimension at the expense of the others may be ineffective in alleviating pain.

Diagnosis, assessment, and evaluation

Diagnosis

This refers to observing that pain is occurring. Diagnosis of pain in children is complicated by the following facts.

- Younger children may lack the necessary abstract conceptual ability to express it.
- Young children may lack the verbal capacity to express pain.
- Many children, particularly in ACT/RCPCH categories III and IV, are developmentally delayed and may be unable to verbalize.
- Children's experience is often reported by parents or other carers, who may be affected by cultural assumptions such as:
  - children do not suffer pain as intensely as adults;
  - children can and should tolerate pain well;
  - children are vulnerable to the adverse effects of painkillers, such that it is better for them to be in pain than risk toxicity.
- The objective signs of pain are the same as those of other causes of distress, such as anxiety, leading observers to conclude that pain is not the cause.

Where there is doubt, it is generally better to assume a child is in pain and treat appropriately, rather than risk allowing them to experience unnecessary discomfort. This can be achieved by:

- recognizing that a child's experience of pain is at least as intense as that of an adult;
- as a default, accepting the word of a parent, nurse, or other carer who knows the child well when they suggest the child may be in pain;
- carefully observing a child's behaviour or using behaviour-based observational skills routinely (see ➜ Chapter 5);
- asking the question 'would I be in pain if this were occurring to me?'

It is rare for families or carers deliberately to overstate a child's pain. If there is doubt, an effective approach is:

- to ask the family member or other carer what behaviour they have observed in the child that leads them to think that they are in pain;
- to record a description of that behaviour carefully;
- to prescribe an appropriate starting dose of an effective analgesic such as an opioid;
- to ask the parent or carer to record over the following week or two whether there has been a reduction in the pain-associated behaviour;
- to review the child a week or two later.

The differential diagnosis here is between pain and other causes of distress, particularly anxiety. Most painkillers are pure analgesics and will have little impact on other causes of distress.

Assessment

Assessment refers to a description of the location, quality, timing, and severity of pain. It can be subject to the same complications in children as diagnosing pain (see ➜ Chapter 5).

Evaluation

This refers to the measurement of pain severity (see ➜ Chapter 5).

Pharmacological treatment of pain

There is a tendency for clinicians to be overcautious in their prescription of strong analgesics, probably for the following reasons.
- Most clinicians are not familiar with most of the available analgesics.
- There are a number of medical cultural myths, including:
  - children feel pain less intensely than adults;
  - children are generally vulnerable to the adverse effects of analgesics;
  - it is unnecessary to use an evidence-based approach in the palliative phase;
  - distraction (e.g. using sucrose solution), anxiolysis (e.g. benzodiazepines), or inducing sleep (e.g. chloral hydrate) are acceptable alternatives to analgesia.
- The 'precautionary principle' is that the small risk of a serious adverse effect should outweigh the certainty of untreated pain.

The result is a tendency for children to receive inadequate analgesia, either by being prescribed medications that are too weak or doses that are too low.

The basic principle underlying appropriate management of pain in palliative care is that the benefits of the proposed treatment, measured in terms of quality of life, should always outweigh its burdens. It is therefore essential to know both the desirable and the adverse effects that are anticipated from a medication.

It is usually possible to find an optimal way of prescribing strong analgesics, so that the risk of adverse effects remains small, while the chance of significant benefit is maximized. This can be achieved by considering:
- which drug to choose;
- the dose of the drug;
- the route of the drug;
- the dosage interval;

These, in turn, depend on variables within the patient:
- age;
- prior medication, particularly analgesics such as opioids;
- concurrent illness;
- what has worked previously in that individual patient;
- nature of the pain, including non-physical factors.

It is quite possible for the same dose of the same drug to be prescribed to two patients who are physically very similar with two very different outcomes (see ➔ Chapter 3, Principle of double effect, p. 24).

It is therefore essential that clinicians demonstrate a rational, and ideally evidence-based, approach to the initiation and escalation of analgesics for pain in palliative care. Departure from this approach risks:
- undertreating pain;
- causing unnecessary adverse effects;
- accusations of professional misconduct such as hastening death.

Management of pain in palliative care differs from pain management in other contexts in the following ways.

• It is usual for there to be more than one source of pain.
• Acute and chronic pain usually coexist.
• Physical pain is complicated by the psychosocial and spiritual context of approaching the end of life.
• Pain is usually gradually increasing in severity. Analgesia in palliative medicine is usually characterized by the need to titrate ever upwards at a carefully considered rate.
• The balance between the benefit of a medication or other intervention against its burden needs to be considered in terms of the immediate quality of life, rather than any long-term considerations.

Palliative pain management in children differs from that in adults for the following reasons.

• Children are often relatively resilient to dose-limiting side effects (e.g. confusion).
• Children needing palliative medicine are rarely ward inpatients. Enabling them to remain in a home or home-like environment has a high priority.
• A high priority must be given to avoiding needles when considering which formulations to choose.
• The range of opioids for which safety information is available in children is relatively limited.
• Palliative medicine in children is usually in collaboration with other paediatricians, and preference often needs to be given to medications that are familiar to paediatricians.

As a result of this, the approach to pain management in children is different in a number of ways.

• Neurolytic procedures are rarely justified.
• Buccal and transdermal preparations are preferred where available.
• Opioids for which evidence of safety and effectiveness is limited should be avoided (such as oxycodone). (Table 4.1 indicates some common errors in prescribing major opioids to children.)

Nevertheless, underlying principles remain the same. Safe and effective management of pain in children is ensured by an understanding of:

• the individual pain;
• the individual child;
• the pathophysiology of pain;
• a graduated approach to pain management.

Table 4.1 Common errors in prescribing major opioids to children

Errors	Consequences
Prescribing major opioids 'as needed' (prn) without background regular major opioids	No background tolerance to adverse effects, particularly drowsiness
	Reduced effectiveness and increased toxicity of prn doses, due to metabolic considerations
	Rapid fluctuations in serum opioid levels, so therapeutic levels reached only occasionally
Wrong dosage interval for oral morphine (e.g. 6-hourly, rather than 4-hourly)	Serum concentrations of opioid fall below therapeutic level, resulting in breakthrough pain
Inappropriate dose of breakthrough opioid relative to regular opioid	The dose of breakthrough opioid should usually be 1/10th to 1/6th of the total daily dose of background regular opioid (see ➲ Chapter 6)
	If the breakthrough dose is too high, tolerance to adverse effects has not developed, and toxicity, particularly drowsiness, will result
	If the dose is too low, it will simply be ineffective because of tolerance to analgesia caused by the background opioid dose
Over-rapid titration of opioids	If the dose of opioids is increased too quickly, there is no time for tolerance to adverse effects to develop. Providing the patient has free access to breakthrough doses of opioid, daily review is usually sufficient and allows titration to be done safely and effectively
Too early conversion to long-acting opioid	Converting to a long-acting opioid should usually be deferred until the opioid requirements have been stable for some days
	Titration of slow-release morphine tablets/granules or fentanyl patches, for example, is constrained, to some extent, by the formulations available
Inaccurate opioid rotation	Opioid rotation is a specialist palliative medicine skill
	Although it is usually possible to exchange one major opioid for another, the exact equivalent dose will depend on a variety of factors, including which drugs they are, how many breakthroughs have been required by the patient, co-prescribed medications, and co-morbidities, particularly renal function
	Furthermore, the phenomenon of incomplete cross-tolerance means that unexpected toxicity can occur, even when substituted with exactly equipotent doses

Modified from WHO Guidelines for analgesic drug therapy. *Cancer Pain Relief and Palliative Care in Children*. Geneva: WHO/IASP; 1998.

WHO pain guidelines

The WHO analgesic ladder originally treated minor opioids, such as codeine, as a separate step. The ladder has recently been revised in recognition that many minor opioids are weak and unreliable, and that a low dose of stronger, more reliable opioids is safer and more effective[3] (Fig. 4.1).

Analgesics for mild pain

Simple analgesia such as:
- paracetamol (= 'acetaminophen' in North America);
- NSAIDs.

Analgesics for moderate to severe pain

Major opioids such as:
- morphine (first line);
- diamorphine;
- fentanyl;
- oxycodone;
- methadone;
- hydromorphone.

Evidence for pethidine in PPM indicates that the risk outweighs the benefit.
  Oxycodone is little different from morphine in its effects.

Opioids should be given 'as needed' for moderate pain and 'around the clock' for severe pain.

	Step 1 Mild pain	Step 2 Moderate pain	Step 3 Severe pain
Drugs	Simple analgesics	Opioids	Opioids
Breakthrough dose	As indicated	0.1mg/kg OME 1–4 hrly	1/10 to 1/6 of total daily background dose, given 1–4 hrly
Background dose	None	Usually none	Starting dose 1mg/kg/24h OME, then increased as determined by breakthrough requirements

Fig. 4.1 WHO pain ladder.
Modified from World Health Organization (2012). WHO guidelines on the pharmacological treatment of persisting pain in children with medical illnesses. www.who.int.

The dangers of codeine
- Is a prodrug for morphine, converted to the active drug by the enzyme CYP2D6.
- WHO no longer recommends codeine in children because:
  - it is a poor prodrug. Only 10% of the drug is converted into morphine in most patients;
  - it is highly inconsistent. There is considerable inter-ethnic variability in the levels of CYP2D6, with between 1% and 30% of individuals within certain ethnic groups not having the enzyme;
  - it works poorly in many children. CYP2D6 levels are low in children (1% in the fetus, 25% in children under 5 years), leading to poor or absent analgesic effects;
  - it is dangerous in others. Some children are hyper-metabolizers and can develop severe opioid toxicity.[3]

Adjuvants
At all steps, an adjuvant should be introduced as soon as the nature of the pain is clear. Adjuvants could include the following.
- For neuropathic pain, anticonvulsants (e.g. gabapentin, carbamazepine), antidepressants (particularly amitriptyline), and NMDA (N-methyl D-aspartate) receptor antagonists (such as methadone and ketamine).
- For bone pain, NSAIDs, bisphosphonates (e.g. pamidronate), and radiotherapy.
- For muscle spasm, muscle relaxants such as benzodiazepine, baclofen, tizanidine, and botulinum toxin.
- For cerebral irritation, anxiolytics such as benzodiazepines or phenobarbital.
- Steroids can be useful in managing inflammatory-mediated pain or pain mediated by oedema round a tumour.
- Chemotherapy. Some chemotherapeutic agents, particularly oral etoposide and vincristine, can reduce the size of a tumour enough to relieve symptoms, without themselves causing major side effects.

'Golden rules'
- Always use oral formulations where possible.
- Use appropriate adjuvants at all stages.
- Major opioids should never be prescribed solely 'as needed'. They should always accompany background major opioids given regularly.

Summary of pain: introduction

- Pain is a subjective and multidimensional phenomenon.
- Diagnosis, assessment, and evaluation of pain are all complicated in children by the range of diagnoses and developmental levels, and by cultural influences.
- Management of pain in palliative care overlaps with, but is different from, management of acute or chronic pain.
- Management of pain in children overlaps with, but is distinct from, management of pain in adults.
- The basic principles of management of pain in palliative care of adults with cancer can be extrapolated reasonably to the care of children with life-limiting conditions.
- The WHO pain ladder is the basis of managing pain in palliative care for children.
- The nature of the paediatric specialty means that the implementation of this approach needs to be modified to make it appropriate for children.

References

1. Task Force on Taxonomy of the International Association for the Study of Pain IASP (1994). Part III: pain terms, a current list with definitions and notes on usage. In: Merskey, H. and Bogduk, N., editors. *Classification of chronic pain*, second edition, pp. 209–14. IASP Press, Seattle.
2. McCaffery, M. and Moss, F. (1968). [Nursing intervention for bodily pain.] *Sogo Kango* 3 (2), 49–58.
3. World Health Organization (2012). *WHO guidelines on the pharmacological treatment of persisting pain in children with medical illnesses.* Available at: ℬ www.who.int.

Chapter 5

Pain evaluation

Introduction

Pain is a subjective phenomenon. It is different for each individual who experiences it and, for any individual, will depend on a multiplicity of factors, including its cause, context, and meaning. The degree of tissue damage is only one factor amongst many that contribute to perception of a painful experience. Pain is modulated by complex neurological, biochemical, and psychological influences at many different levels from the periphery to the cortex. Even the 'wiring' of the system itself is subject to change, particularly during childhood. This may result from previous pain experience. The sensation of pain is therefore influenced by innumerable factors, not only at the time of the stimulus, but during the individual's prior experience.

A distinction is sometimes made between 'assessment' and 'measurement' of pain. Measurement refers specifically to quantification of pain, i.e. how severe it is. Assessment describes the broader diagnosis and estimation of a pain experience. Scales that simply quantify pain may not also adequately describe it.

Appropriate tools can report aspects of pain experience (Box 5.1). Across childhood, changing developmental levels mean it may be necessary to select from a range of tools in order to assess and measure pain effectively. All children receiving analgesics should ideally be subject to routine assessment of their pain. That this is not usually done is partly a result of the traditionally low priority given to pain in children, but the problem is compounded by scales that are:

• difficult to use;
• uninteresting to children;
• unwieldy for staff.

Selecting the right scale is important, but a scale that is highly validated and eminently suitable for research may be simply too cumbersome for day-to-day clinical use.

Box 5.1 QUEST approach to managing pain in a child

• Question the child.
• Use pain-rating tools.
• Evaluate behaviour.
• Sensitize parents (i.e. ask them to report the child's pain).
• Take action (i.e. prescribe appropriate analgesic intervention).

Characteristics of a pain scale

The ideal pain scale should have the following characteristics.
- Practical. It must capture a child's imagination and be fun to use, as well as simple and quick for staff to administer.
- Appropriately validated. A scale should measure the right phenomenon. Scales measuring physiological responses to pain do not distinguish between pain and anxiety. Since the purpose of a pain scale is to decide on analgesic therapy, a pain scale should measure the symptom that can be treated using analgesics.
- Appropriately applied. Some pain scales have been developed for specific clinical situations. It should not be assumed they will be equally valid in others. For example, scales measuring acute pain are unlikely to be equally valid in measuring chronic pain. This is particularly true of scales relying on behavioural observations, which are often based on patterns derived during specific procedures.
- Developmentally appropriate. No single pain scale is valid across all age groups. Since pain is subjective, and subjective experience needs to be reported by an individual, it is essential that a scale should allow the child to self-report where possible.
- Culturally appropriate. Because pain is reported as a subjective phenomenon, the use of language is potentially very important. The use of culturally specific terms (e.g. 'ouchie' in the United States (US)) limits usefulness. Scales relying on facial expression should either be racially neutral or be available for different racial groups.

Special groups

Neonates and infants
Generally unsatisfactory, but important, measures:
- physiological measures of autonomic function;
- biochemical measures (cortisol, endorphins);
- behavioural measures (nature of cry, facial expression, flailing of arms and legs).

Children with developmental delay
- Important, as pain is a consistent feature.
- Many children are capable of a degree of expression of subjective pain.
- Parents or carers become expert in recognizing pain behaviours and should be believed when they report it.
- Some pain behaviours are common to many children and have been described and correlated with objective measures.
- Therapeutic trial of analgesic may be necessary to demonstrate the presence or absence of pain.

Classification of pain scales

There are, in fact, many different pain scales available for children. They match this ideal to a greater or lesser extent. They fall into five categories:
- visual analogue self-report scales;
- descriptive self-report scales;
- objective measures of pain;
- behavioural measures;
- multidimensional pain scales.

Self-report scales

Visual analogue self-report scales

The most direct means of assessing pain in a child may simply be to ask 'how much does it hurt?'. Providing there is an appropriate tool to quantify it, most children have the necessary abstract ability to respond to this. There are many such tools.

Under 6 years old

Faces scale

A self-report scale comprising a range of expressions from smiling broadly to crying inconsolably.
- Strengths:
  - attractive;
  - simple;
  - quick to administer.
- Weaknesses:
  - faces might equally express mood, rather than pain;
  - expressions depict response to acute, rather than chronic, pain.

The Oucher

Refinement of the Faces scale, using photographs of real faces linked to a numerical visual analogue scale of 0–100.
- Strengths:
  - well-designed;
  - rigorously validated;
  - can be used over a wide range of ages, due to a combination of photos and numerical index;
  - race-appropriate alternatives are available.
- Weakness: expressions are those of acute pain, rather than chronic.

Poker chip tool

This uses red plastic poker chips representing 'pieces of hurt', allowing children to choose from 1 ('a little bit of hurt') to 4 ('a lot of hurt').
- Strengths:
  - very attractive to children;
  - simple;
  - widely culturally applicable;
  - has been validated.
- Weakness: limited range of responses available.

Colour scales

An outline of a child's body that a child can colour in using pens or crayons. The child first selects which colours will represent 'worst hurt' and which represent 'no hurt at all'.
- Strengths:
  - quickly engages a child's interest;
  - fun to complete;
  - allows expression of feelings of pain;
  - allows the child to describe the exact site of pain.
- Weakness relatively poorly validated.

Other scales
There are many other variations on the theme of a visual analogue scale, including:
- a glasses scale;
- a ladder scale;
- a line scale.

Six years to adolescence
Many of the analogue scales designed for younger children can be used in this age group as well. Scales developed in adults become increasingly appropriate, as the child approaches adolescence. Most are based on a visual analogue scale.
- Strengths:
  - well-validated in adults;
  - often validated in children;
  - simple to use;
  - quick to administer.
- Weaknesses:
  - can only measure one dimension of pain at a time (usually intensity). A broader assessment can be made using a visual analogue scale to quantify an additional dimension such as 'the degree of unpleasantness of pain';
  - may be less valid for chronic pain due to functional habituation (a child may simply forget what it was like not to be in pain).

Descriptive self-report scales
Since pain is a subjective phenomenon, the child's own description of the nature and severity of their pain is ultimately what needs to be assessed. There are many descriptive self-report scales.
- Strengths:
  - accesses subjective experience of pain;
  - based on well-validated concept in adults;
  - further validated in children.
- Weaknesses:
  - pain descriptors are known to be influenced by age;
  - labour-intensive, making it difficult to use in clinical situations;
  - original descriptors derived from acute pain, but validated in children with chronic pain.

Objective and behavioural measures of pain

Objective measures of pain

The phrase appears inherently contradictory, since pain is a subjective experience. Objective assessments can be made, however, of the effect of pain on some measurable physiological parameter.

Strengths
- Easy for staff to carry out routinely.
- Independent of developmental stage or capacity to communicate.

Weaknesses
- Take no account of emotional, psychological, or spiritual aspects of pain.
- Do not distinguish between pain and other causes of distress.
- Do not allow subjective report of pain experience.

These weaknesses mean that purely physiological parameters are no longer acceptable assessments for children's pain. However, they remain important where there is no alternative, e.g. in some neonatal contexts.

Physiological parameters may, however, add to the discriminatory power of other scales.

Behavioural measures of pain

Pain is always associated with meaning and fear, which has been termed 'catastrophizing'. In children under 3 years, communication of that fear is not primarily verbal but uses non-verbal behaviour patterns. Behavioural scales formalize observation of behaviour patterns associated with pain. They allow interpretation of a child's communication of subjective experience. They are not therefore objective measures, although they rely on observation. Since 'body language' remains a feature of communication at all ages, all groups of children and adults (particularly those with impaired cognitive function such as cerebral palsy or neurodegenerative conditions) may also use these.

Strengths
- Allow interpretation of subjective pain experience by the observer.
- Do not depend on the child's willingness to participate.
- Potentially can be used for most developmental stages.
- By identifying appropriate behaviour patterns, can be equally valid for acute and chronic pain.
- By identifying appropriate behaviour patterns, can be used for children with impaired cognition or ability to communicate.

Weaknesses
- Often labour-intensive and unwieldy to use in clinical practice.
- Appropriate application is determined by derivation of behaviour patterns. For example, behaviour patterns associated with pain due to procedures may not be seen in chronic cancer pain.
- Some behaviours are age-dependent.

Further reading

Baker, C.M. and Wong, D.L. (1987). Q.U.E.S.T.: a process of pain assessment in children (continuing education credit). *Orthop. Nurs.* **6** (1), 11–21.

Beyer, J.E., Denyes, M.J., and Villarruel, A.M. (1992). The creation, validation, and continuing development of the Oucher: a measure of pain intensity in children. *J. Pediatr. Nurs.* **7** (5), 335–46.

Gauvain-Piquard, A., Rodary, C., Rezvani, A., and Serbouti, S. (1999). The development of the DEGR(R): A scale to assess pain in young children with cancer. *Eur. J. Pain* **3** (2), 165–76.

Hain, R.D. (1997). Pain scales in children: a review. *Palliat. Med.* **11** (5), 341–50.

Hicks, C.L., von Baeyer, C.L., Spafford, P.A., van Korlaar, I., and Goodenough, B. (2001). The Faces Pain Scale–Revised: toward a common metric in pediatric pain measurement. *Pain* **93** (2), 173–83.

Hunt, A., Goldman, A., Seers, K., *et al.* (2004). Clinical validation of the paediatric pain profile. *Dev. Med. Child Neurol.* **46**. 9–18.

Parkerson, H.A., Noel, M., Page, M.G., Fuss, S., Katz, J., and Asmundson, G.J. (2013). Factorial validity of the English-language version of the Pain Catastrophizing Scale—child version. *J. Pain* **14** (11), 1383–9.

Chapter 6

Pain: step 3, major opioids

Introduction

Drugs at step 3 are considered major opioids (or sometimes 'strong opioids' or 'opioids for severe pain'). The choice of drugs available on this step is greater than on any of the others. Opioids can be considered as:
- naturally occurring ('opiates' such as morphine, diamorphine (heroin));
- synthetic (fentanyl, buprenorphine);
- semi-synthetic (hydromorphone, pethidine (meperidine)).

While the mechanism of action of opioids is similar, they may have distinct properties with respect to:
- action at opioid receptor subtypes (μ_1, μ_2, delta, kappa) and action at non-opioid receptors (NMDA, substance P, etc.);
- potency;
- adverse effects profile;
- cost;
- formulation;
- availability;
- metabolism.

All of these should be taken into consideration when selecting the appropriate opioid for the situation. There are some general guiding principles (see also Table 4.1).
- Oral morphine is the major opioid of choice for first-line treatment because:
  - the research base in adults is strong and, though weaker in children, is stronger than for other opioids;
  - morphine is usually well tolerated;
  - morphine is usually effective, irrespective of the cause for pain.
- Major opioids should never be prescribed 'as needed', unless there is also regular background major opioid analgesia. There is no need for two major opioids prescribed 'regularly' and 'as needed' to be of the same class.
- Major opioids should never be prescribed regularly without also making available 'breakthrough' doses as needed.
- The breakthrough dose should always be between one-tenth and one-sixth of the total daily dose, when standardized to 'oral morphine equivalence' (OME) (Box 6.1).
- The phenomena of tolerance, dependence, and addiction are distinct and should not be confused.
  - Tolerance: shift in the dose–response curve, such that a greater dose of the drug is required for the same effect. This refers equally to desirable and adverse effects.
  - Dependence: physical changes that occur, often at receptor level, during long-term treatment with a drug that mean it should not be discontinued abruptly.
  - Addiction: complex physical, psychosocial, and spiritual phenomenon in which the individual is unable to function without the drug.

Box 6.1 Oral morphine equivalence

- OME is the observation that the potency of major opioids can be described in terms of each other by comparison with oral morphine (the 'standard unit' of opioid potency).
  - For example, oral diamorphine is ~1.5 times as potent as oral morphine, while oral hydromorphine is between 5 and 7.5 times the potency of oral morphine. Thus, the OME of oral diamorphine is 1.5, while that of oral hydromorphone would be between 5 and 7.5.
- OME has largely been extrapolated from data in adults but, in practice, seems to work well in children.
- There is very little evidence regarding equianalgesic doses using drugs by different routes. As a rule of thumb, bioavailability via intravenous (iv), subcutaneous (sc), transcutaneous, or transmucosal routes is considered to be twice that of oral bioavailability for most major opioids.

Prescribing major opioids

In prescribing major opioids appropriately, the following should be taken into consideration.[1]

- Which drug?
- At what dose?
- By what route?

Incomplete cross-tolerance

- Tolerance to different effects of a medication can develop at different rates in a single individual.
  - Tolerance to the analgesic effects of morphine occurs very slowly.
  - Tolerance to drowsiness develops within 2 or 3 days.
  - Tolerance to constipation does not develop at all.
- This is also true for different opioids, particularly those of different classes.
- Tolerance to analgesia may occur more slowly than tolerance to adverse effects.
- This means that changing to a different major opioid ('rotation' or 'substitution') can provide relief from some adverse effects (such as neuroexcitability) by allowing a reduction in OME opioid dose with no loss of analgesia.

Morphine

Oral morphine is the major opioid of choice in palliative medicine. It is the archetypal major opioid.

Strengths

- Powerfully analgesic in most pain.
- Usually well tolerated.
- Tolerance to its analgesic effects develops slowly and is easily managed by increasing the dose.
- Tolerance to some adverse effects develops quickly (especially drowsiness, which typically resolves within 48h of commencing morphine, with no modification in the dose).
- Evidence base in adult palliative medicine is excellent, and in children very good.
- Available in slow- and immediate-release oral formulations, as well as parenteral ones.

Weaknesses

- Constipation: tolerance does not develop to constipation, and, in most cases, laxatives should be automatically co-prescribed. Movicol® or a combination of stimulant and softening laxatives are suitable. Lactulose alone is not recommended.
- Respiratory depression: much feared, but extremely rare.
- Fears of addiction: the risk is slight, but the fears are real, and should be anticipated and pre-emptively addressed.
- Can be associated by the child and/or family with 'terminal phase' and accelerated progress towards death.

Alternative, non-morphine opioids

Use of non-morphine opioids in palliative care is a specialist skill, and advice should be sought from the paediatric (or, if there is none, adult) palliative medicine team.

Diamorphine

- OME 1.5.
- Formulations: parenteral, oral, buccal.
- Advantages over morphine: more highly soluble, so can be given buccally, and high doses can be dissolved in relatively small volumes.
- Disadvantages: as diamorphine rapidly cleaved to morphine after administration, not suitable for rotation/substitution.
- Evidence base: as for morphine.

Fentanyl

- OME 150.
- Available formulations: transdermal patch, parenteral, transmucosal (immediate-release).
- Advantages over morphine:
  - complementary receptor profile, so works well alongside morphine breakthrough;
  - available as a 72-hourly transdermal patch;
  - probably less constipating;
  - of a different class, so suitable for opioid rotation/substitution.
- Disadvantages:
  - patches unsuitable for titration phase.
- Evidence base in children: good.
- Evidence base in adults: very good.

Buprenorphine

- OME 60.
- Available formulations: transdermal patch, sublingual.
- Advantages over morphine:
  - available as a transdermal patch;
  - probably less constipating;
  - patch doses encompass steps 2 and 3, so can replace codeine;
  - of a different class, so suitable for opioid rotation/substitution.
- Disadvantages: incidence of poor tolerability (nausea, vomiting, respiratory depression) higher than morphine, more difficult to reverse in overdosage as partial agonist.
- Evidence base in children: poor in palliative medicine; adequate in acute pain.
- Evidence base in adults: good.

Tramadol

- A derivative of codeine.
- OME 0.2, but effective potency greater than this due to non-opioid analgesic effects via modulation of GABAergic, noradrenergic, and serotonergic systems.

- No evidence of specific benefit in neuropathic pain, though NMDA antagonism has been suggested.
- Very poorly tolerated in a minority of patients due primarily to hypotension.
- Evidence for safety and effectiveness in acute pain in children.
- No evidence of effectiveness and safety in chronic or palliative care pain.

The role of tramadol in paediatric palliative care has yet to be determined and is probably limited. It is not recommended by the WHO but, in practice, is valuable in countries where there is no access to fast-acting opioids.

Methadone
- OME variable.
- Available formulations: oral, parenteral.
- Advantages over morphine:
  - probably has additional non-opioid effects (particularly NMDA blockade, giving adjuvant effect in neuropathic pain and potentially in bone pain);
  - different class from morphine, so suitable for rotation/substitution.
- Disadvantages:
  - difficult to calculate conversion, as OME variable depending on dose;
  - distributes to body fat, which becomes saturated, so theoretical risk of sudden fatal increase in serum concentration with no change in administered dose;
- Evidence base in children: many case series, some in palliative medicine.
- Evidence base in adults: very good.

Hydromorphone
- OME 5–7.5.
- Available formulations: oral, parenteral.
- Advantages over morphine:
  - few in the UK; in countries without access to diamorphine, provides an alternative solution for dissolving high doses;
  - structurally similar to morphine, but probably different enough for effective rotation/substitution.
- Disadvantages:
  - slightly more expensive in most places.
- Evidence base in children: good, though most not in palliative medicine.
- Evidence base in adults: very good.

At what dose?

The dose and route should be selected on the basis of the phase of management. There are three phases of opioid prescription:[1]

- initiation;
- titration;
- maintenance.

Initiation

An appropriate starting dose can be arrived at by:

- calculating on basis of weight; or
- converting from existing opioid requirements on basis of OME (i.e. opioid rotation/substitution; see ➔ Chapter 6, Alternative, non-morphine opioids, pp. 51–2).

For all prescriptions, it is imperative to ensure:

- use of regular immediate-release preparation initially;
- correct prescription of regular and breakthrough doses (Table 4.1) (the breakthrough dose should be 1/10 or 1/6 of the total daily dose OME, given at least 4-hourly, as needed);
- the child and family know that breakthrough is available quickly, when needed.

Titration

The need for major opioid analgesia is matched against the intensity of pain over a period of days by:

- review of the need for breakthrough over a 48h period;
- recalculation of the regular dose by adding to it the total daily requirements of breakthrough;
- recalculation of breakthrough, so that it remains the same proportion of 1/10 or 1/6 of the total;
- repeated review after 48h.

Maintenance

Once pain has been matched by analgesia, such that changes to the dose have become infrequent, convenience can be improved by switching to a long-acting formulation such as:

- slow-release morphine;
- transdermal patch (fentanyl, buprenorphine);
- syringe driver (diamorphine, fentanyl).

Even during the maintenance phase, breakthrough doses of an immediate-release formulation (ideally oral, e.g. morphine, methadone) should continue to be made available in the same proportion, i.e. 1/10 or 1/6 of the total daily dose OME.

By what route?

The most appropriate route is determined by several factors.

Child's preference

Whatever the science behind choosing the right route, no medication will work if the child finds it unpleasant to take. While most children prefer syrups to tablets, and prefer the oral route to others, those are *by no means universal. The preferences of the individual child* must dictate the route, where possible.

In order of general acceptability to children, available routes are:
* enteral (oral or gastrostomy);
* transcutaneous;
* buccal (or other transmucosal such as sublingual or nasal spray);
* sc;
* iv;
* rectal.

NB. The intramuscular (im) route has not been acceptable in children for many years.

Whether it is the initiation, titration, or maintenance phase

(See ➲ Chapter 6, At what dose?, p. 53.)

The enteral route is flexible. Enteral medications are often ideal for initiation and titration, but are unsuitable for maintenance, as they typically need to be given every few hours to maintain serum concentrations. Transcutaneous patches are ideal in the maintenance phase but usually inappropriate for initiation or titration, because the dose is not easily altered.

Simplicity

The subcutaneous route avoids the need for repeated attempts at cannulation associated with the intravenous (or the risks of sepsis associated with central venous lines) and does not need medical supervision. Subcutaneous is the preferred route outside the acute ward environment.

Urgency

Where rapid control of escalating pain is needed, the parenteral route using a continuous driver is usually the most effective.

Biotransformation

Particularly hepatic metabolism, which can be bypassed by use of the buccal or other parenteral route.

Physical characteristics of the drug

* *Lipid solubility* will determine whether the drug will cross the skin (and possibly the mucous membrane).
* *Water solubility* will determine whether it will dissolve in saliva (important in buccal or nasal use if the drug is to access the mucous membrane) or dissolve in small volumes of water for infusion.
* Vesicant properties (whether it will be painful to give).

What formulations of the drug are available?

For example, in the UK, methadone is only easily available orally, so is not always an option, even in clinical situations where its pharmacology suggests it would be ideal. Oxycodone, on the other hand, has no pharmacological advantages over morphine and is a great deal more expensive, but it is available as a suppository.

Specific clinical situations

- Active vomiting contraindicates the oral route.
- Neutropenia contraindicates the rectal route.
- Skin sepsis, allergies, or local reactions may contraindicate routes involving the skin.
- Bleeding diathesis may contraindicate the subcutaneous route.

Practical issues

Buccal medications

Why?

The buccal route entails dissolving an opioid in a small volume of water for injection and giving the solution between the child's gum and cheek using a small syringe with no needle. It offers a number of theoretical advantages over other routes:

- easy to give, so minimizes delay in administering breakthrough;
- does not require the child to be able to cooperate (cf. sublingual or nasal);
- does not involve needles;
- often familiar to families, as it is used for seizure medications;
- small volume and rapid absorption mean the route can often be used, even for bitter medications;
- rapidly absorbed into blood;
- bypasses liver metabolism.

What dose?

Transmucosal routes avoid first-pass metabolism.[2] In animal studies, pharmacokinetics of transmucosal fentanyl is the same as iv fentanyl.[3] In humans, bioavailability of fentanyl is significantly higher by the transmucosal route than by the oral.[4] In children, bioavailability of 100% is usually assumed (i.e. the same as parenteral routes such as intravenous or subcutaneous, but twice that of enteral routes such as oral or gastrostomy). In practice, bioavailability might be less than that, because not all the drug is absorbed, so a proportion might be swallowed. Any such under-dosing in practice can be resolved with appropriate titration.

Morphine or diamorphine?

- Anecdotally, both have their supporters, but diamorphine offers the benefit of dissolving in particularly small volumes of water for injection.
- Lipid-soluble drugs cross cell membranes well. More water-soluble drugs dissolve in saliva quickly and arrive at the mucosa rapidly. Buccal absorption depends on both.
- Currently, no convincing comparison research evidence.
- Fentanyl (much more highly lipid-soluble than either morphine or diamorphine) is well absorbed by the buccal route in adults.[5]

Changing from patch to driver

Transcutaneous opioid patches become less useful in the face of rapidly changing requirements, as it is not easy to titrate them rapidly. That is particularly likely at the end of life, at a time when the child is unable to tolerate enteral alternatives.

In adults, the recommendation in some places is to commence the syringe driver some time before removing the opioid patch, in order to allow serum concentrations of the new opioid to accumulate. In paediatrics, where the patient is typically pre- or non-verbal and often cared for by teams working in shifts, the risk is that the patch is inadvertently left *in situ*, resulting in a potentially dangerous doubling of the opioid dose.

A safer approach is to:

- calculate the syringe driver dose using OME, as described earlier;
- ensure an appropriate dose of breakthrough opioid is available 1- to 4-hourly in a rapidly acting form such as buccal diamorphine;
- advise parents and staff at the bedside to be particularly aware of the child's need for breakthrough in the next 12h and to have a low threshold for intervening with breakthrough opioid;
- commence the syringe driver and remove the patch at the same time.

In most cases, elimination of the old opioid is more or less matched by accumulation of the new one, so that therapeutic concentrations are maintained throughout the transition. The child has free access to adequate breakthrough for top-up, in case there is breakthrough pain as the two 'cross over'.

References

1. Drake, R., Friedrichsdorf, S.J., and Hain, R.D.W. (2012). Pharmacological approaches to pain. 2: Simple analgesics and opioids. In: Goldman, A., Hain, R., and Liben, S., editors. *Oxford textbook of palliative care for children*, pp. 234–46. Oxford University Press, Oxford.
2. Mystakidou, K., Katsouda, E., Parpa, E., Vlahos, L., and Tsiatas, M.L. (2006). Oral transmucosal fentanyl citrate: overview of pharmacological and clinical characteristics. *Drug Deliv.* **13**, 269–76.
3. Little, A.A., Krotscheck, U., Boothe, D.M., and Erb, H.N. (2008 Fall). Pharmacokinetics of buccal mucosal administration of fentanyl in a carboxymethylcellulose gel compared with IV administration in dogs. *Vet. Ther.* **9**, 201–11.
4. Darwish, M., Kirby, M., Robertson, P., Jr., Tracewell, W., and Jiang, J.G. (2007). Absolute and relative bioavailability of fentanyl buccal tablet and oral transmucosal fentanyl citrate. *J. Clin. Pharmacol.* **47**, 343–50.
5. Grape, S., Schug, S.A., Lauer, S., and Schug, B.S. (2010). Formulations of fentanyl for the management of pain. *Drugs* **70** (1), 57–72.

Adjuvants

Introduction

- An adjuvant is not analgesic but is capable of relieving pain in certain specific pain situations. Selection of an appropriate adjuvant is a key element of a rational and evidence-based approach to management of pain in children. It depends on diagnosis of the type of pain (see ⤳ Chapter 7, Diagnosis of pain, pp. 59–60).
- Choice of an adjuvant is on the basis of the nature of pain, rather than its intensity. Suitable adjuvants should be considered at all steps of the WHO pain ladder.
- Adjuvants are more specific, but not necessarily more potent, than analgesics. For example:
  - amitriptyline is more specific to neuropathic pain than morphine; *and*
  - neuropathic pain is less likely to be sensitive to morphine than other forms of pain; *but*
  - the effectiveness of morphine is such that it is probably more likely to produce a beneficial effect than amitriptyline, even in neuropathic pain.
- Classic examples of adjuvants are anticonvulsants and antidepressants for relief of neuropathic pain.
- NSAIDs are usually considered adjuvants for bone pain but are, in fact, analgesic in their own right.

Diagnosis of pain

Selection of a suitable adjuvant depends critically on recognizing the nature of the pain syndrome to be treated. A systematic approach to evaluation of pain, including its history, physical signs, and, where necessary, investigation, is essential (see ➲ Chapter 5). Box 7.1 gives a useful mnemonic for taking a pain history.

There are many different ways to classify pain. For the purposes of selecting adjuvant medications, the most useful is the following.

Neuropathic pain

This is characterized by:
- disordered sensation (numbness, allodynia, dysaesthesia, hyperaesthesia);
- a plausible nerve distribution, such as a dermatome, or, in the case of sympathetic-mediated pain, a vascular distribution.

Central or thalamic pain, resulting from direct damage to the thalamus, is a special example of neuropathic pain that may be difficult to identify and treat.

Bone pain

Characteristically:
- focal, deep-seated, intense;
- occurring in the context of conditions causing metastasis or osteoporotic fracture;
- where these are complicated by a pathological fracture or joint dislocation, may present as incident pain.

Muscle spasm or colic

Typically:
- intense but short-lived;
- often occurs in children without the cognitive or verbal ability to identify its location;
- between painful episodes, the child may be pain-free.

Box 7.1 PQRST mnemonic for taking an adequate pain history

Using this, it should be possible to make a diagnosis of the likely pain syndrome and select the appropriate adjuvant accordingly.
- Precipitating and relieving factors.
- Quality of the pain (i.e. neuropathic? bone pain? muscle spasm?).
- Radiation of pain.
- Severity of pain (use appropriate pain assessment tool).
- Timing of pain.

Cerebral irritation

Typically:
- follows acute brain injury such as perinatal asphyxia or intracerebral bleed;
- caused by amplification of pain and anxiety;
- occurs in the neonatal period but may also result from trauma, infection, or malignancy in older children.

Incident pain

Incident pain is breakthrough pain from an intermittent cause (e.g. fracture), rather than from inadequate background analgesia. It can be difficult to treat, and specialist paediatric (or, if that is not available, adult) palliative medicine advice should be sought.

Adjuvants for neuropathic pain

Anticonvulsants (especially sodium valproate, carbamazepine, gabapentin, or pregabalin)

Since seizures and pain both result from undesirable firing of neurons, it is understandable that anticonvulsants are effective in neuropathic-type pain.

Antidepressants

Particularly amitriptyline. Generally speaking, the older tricyclic antidepressants, such as amitriptyline, are more effective in managing neuropathic pain than later ones or antidepressants, such as duloxetine, which are of a different class. Amitriptyline also has sedative and anticholinergic properties that may be of additional benefit in symptom control. By the same token, however, these may limit its use in some patients. The anti-neuropathic dose of amitriptyline is approximately a fifth the antidepressant dose. Its analgesic effects are often seen within a few days.

Lidocaine patches

Lidocaine patches are believed to provide a local effect through transdermal absorption.[1] Experience with their use in children is limited, but anecdotal reports suggest they may be of particular value in pain caused by tissues of neurogenic origin, such as neurofibromas, neuroblastoma, or Ewing's sarcoma, particularly where these are superficial. The patches should be applied directly over the painful lesion.

NMDA antagonists

The NMDA receptors are involved in neuronal plasticity, i.e. the accommodation of a neural system to ongoing or repeated pain. The NMDA antagonist/class of medications can relieve neuropathic pain through interference with this mechanism.

Methadone

Methadone is, in principle, an ideal agent for relief of neuropathic pain, since it combines the properties of major opioid and NMDA antagonists. There is accumulating evidence of its safety and effectiveness in children,[2] and it is generally well tolerated. In adults, regular methadone can result in saturation of body fat in such a way that there is a sudden increase in serum levels after a few days of treatment. In most adult palliative care units, therefore, it is only commenced on inpatients. This has severely limited its usefulness in children, whose palliative care is usually delivered in the home. It is unclear whether this 'secondary peak phenomenon' occurs in children, but it seems prudent to restrict methadone use to breakthrough pain or to the small number of children whose palliative care is to be managed in an inpatient unit.

Ketamine

The pain-relieving effects of ketamine can occur in doses much lower than those used for anaesthesia. Ketamine has long been used in children, and its safety profile is well known. It is also known to result in frightening alterations in perception, particularly auditory hallucinations, and, for that reason, should be used with caution in children. A benefit of ketamine is that its oral bioavailability is very high, so that it can be given enterally.

Steroids

Because of their protean effects, steroids can be adjuvants for a wide range of pain conditions. Where nerve pain is caused by pressure (e.g. due to tumour), steroids can reduce oedema temporarily and help secure analgesia in the short term. The adverse effects of steroids mean that their use should usually be restricted to 2 or 5 days at a time, but this can be at high dose.

Neurolytic procedures

Neurolytic procedures (e.g. epidural anaesthetic, local regional anaesthesia, coeliac axis nerve block) can be highly effective. The necessity for a hospital admission and a needle means they are much less commonly used in PPM than in the adult specialty. It can be difficult to provide analgesia without also impacting on motor function. Consultation with paediatric anaesthetic colleagues should be considered early, particularly when pain is focal and unrelieved by systemic measures.

Adjuvants for bone pain

NSAIDs

NSAIDs are not technically adjuvants, since they have analgesic properties in their own right. They do, however, appear to have a specific role in managing bone pain. NSAIDs suppress production of inflammatory and pain mediators such as prostaglandins, thus reducing the sensation of pain and the cause of it. NSAIDs have a wide adverse effect profile, including gastrointestinal side effects, potential worsening of bronchospasm, and impacts on renal blood flow. In paediatric palliative care, an individual judgement should be made of the risk of severe adverse effects against potential benefit. Gastrointestinal side effects can be attenuated by combined use of a proton pump inhibitor.

Steroids

Steroids can reduce bone pain through reduction in inflammation and oedema around malignant microdeposits. They should be used with caution (see ➲ Chapter 7, Adjuvants for neuropathic pain, Steroids, p. 62).

Radiotherapy

For bone pain caused by metastatic deposits, radiotherapy can provide dramatic and long-lasting relief from pain. This is particularly true of radiosensitive malignancies (e.g. leukaemias, Ewing's sarcoma), but good results can be obtained, even in radioresistant disease (e.g. osteosarcoma). One visit to hospital for a single fraction of radiotherapy may be all that is necessary. Radiotherapy opinion should be sought whenever bone pain is caused by malignancy.

Bisphosphonates

Bisphosphonates are pyrophosphate analogues that inhibit lytic activity of the bone cortex by osteoclasts. Bisphosphonates have been used for some years[3] in adults with bone metastases. It is becoming clear[4] that they have a role in the much wider range of causes for bone pain seen in children. Evidence currently suggests that they are well tolerated by most children. Current guidelines suggest that iv pamidronate should be given at 3-monthly intervals, and that the initial dose should be given over 3 days as an inpatient. Subsequent doses can be given at home if the necessary nursing and medical support are available. While their analgesic effects may be apparent within only a few weeks, patients should normally receive them for at least a year, before a definitive assessment of their effectiveness can be made.

Orthopaedic interventions

Where there is a specific bony injury or abnormality (such as hip dislocation, pathological fracture, or scoliosis), an orthopaedic opinion should always be sought. While, for many children, definitive corrective surgery may not be appropriate or even possible, there may be other interventions that can help. These may range from constructing pseudarthrosis to intra-articular injections of local anaesthetic and steroid.

Neurolytic procedures

These can be effective, particularly if a single limb is the source for pain. They are uncomfortable and usually require hospital admission, both of which limit their usefulness in children (see ➲ Chapter 7, Adjuvants for neuropathic pain, pp. 61–2).

Adjuvants for muscle spasm

The term 'spasm' is used to mean at least three related, but distinct, phenomena:
- intermittent, intense, but short-lived, contraction of muscles;
- chronic hypertonicity of muscles;
- seizure-like activity without changes in the encephalogram (EEG).

All three may occur in a single patient, particularly those in ACT/RCPCH groups III and IV.
- Seizure-like spasms may not be painful or distressing. Overtreatment may result in unnecessary adverse effects.
- Management of chronic muscle spasm should be in close collaboration with colleagues in neurodisability, community paediatrics, and paediatric neurology. Associated pain may be due to joint deformity and contractures, rather than to muscle spasm itself.
- Acute muscle spasm is characterized by pain that is:
  - severe;
  - short-lived;
  - intermittent.

The main drug interventions available are the following.

Benzodiazepines
- Buccal midazolam is rapidly absorbed and short-acting. It can be administered by parents when acute muscle spasm occurs.
- If buccal midazolam is needed frequently, regular longer-acting benzodiazepines (such as diazepam or lorazepam) may reduce the frequency of spasms.
- The metabolites of diazepam are active and long-lasting but, in children, seem to be well tolerated.

Antispasmodics: baclofen
- Baclofen can reduce the frequency and severity of painful muscle spasms.
- It tends to affect truncal muscle tone disproportionately (can adversely affect posture).
- It can be given orally, parenterally, or via an intrathecal pump with good effect. (This requires input from specialist centres.)
- Baclofen can reduce the seizure threshold and complicate the management of fits.

Other antispasmodics
There are numerous other antispasmodics available through specialist paediatric neurology services, including tizanidine, dantrolene, and cyclobenzaprine.

Botulinum toxin
- Given by local injection into muscle.
- Effects last several weeks.
- Can give an indication of potential benefit from orthopaedic interventions, e.g. tenotomy.
- Effects can accumulate, leading to systemic neurological problems.
- Requires specialist orthopaedic or neurodisability involvement.

Need for teamworking
In managing symptomatic muscle spasm, it is important to collaborate closely with colleagues coordinating seizure medication because:
- some antispasmodics can change seizure threshold and therefore complicate anticonvulsant management;
- some anticonvulsants are also effective antispasmodics, reducing the risk of unnecessary polypharmacy;
- specialist neurology interventions may be effective where palliative care ones have failed (e.g. tizanidine, botulinum toxin).

Adjuvants for cerebral irritation

Cerebral irritation is a form of 'total' pain. It comprises:
- pain from physical causes such as cerebral oedema and cerebral haemorrhage;
- anxiety, exacerbated by an inability to process neurological stimuli and understand their context;
- temporal disorientation and disruption of the sleep/wake cycle;
- reflected anxiety from exhausted and sleep-deprived carers.

Cerebral irritation is caused by acute inflammation.
- Following hypoxic–ischaemic encephalopathy in the neonatal period, treatment should continue for 3–6 months and gradually give way to conventional management of the effects of residual neurological deficit.
- Following acute cerebral trauma or infection, treatment should continue in a similar way.
- Where caused by malignant disease, treatment should continue until death, unless some other intervention, such as palliative chemotherapy or radiotherapy, intervenes.
- Phenobarbital, benzodiazepines, and opioids should be weaned gradually, in order to avoid rebound symptoms.

Suitable adjuvants include the following.
- Phenobarbital. An effective soporific and anxiolytic. It is also a useful anticonvulsant, though its long-term use is restricted by adverse effects. Phenobarbital can be given orally or via parenteral infusion. Although phenobarbital can be given subcutaneously, it cannot be combined with most other medications. It requires a dedicated syringe driver, which may be unacceptable to some families.
- Benzodiazepines. A combination of:
  - long-acting benzodiazepine (e.g. lorazepam, diazepam);
  - immediate- and short-acting (e.g. buccal midazolam) for 'breakthrough' cerebral irritation.
- Opioids. While most children with cerebral irritation cannot express that they are in pain, it seems a reasonable assumption, since the causes of cerebral irritation are also causes for pain (acute brain injury, leptomeningeal metastatic spread, acute inflammation).

Pain syndromes

Central pain

Definition

Is a form of neuropathic pain associated with increasing pain, as the bladder fills or a viscera distends.

Management

- Various drugs have been tried, with mixed results. Evidence currently only based on case studies. The following drugs have been tried:
  - amitriptyline;
  - gabapentin;
  - pregabalin.[5]

Visceral hyperalgesia

Definition

Is a type of neuropathic pain where there is a decrease in the threshold of pain activation from visceral stimulation such as intraluminal distension.

Symptoms

Pain and abdominal distension in children after feeds or at particular times of the day.

Management

- Venting of gastrostomy.
- Slowing down of feeds or reduction of feed strengths.
- Surgery for gastro-oesophageal reflux has been identified as a risk factor for developing these pains.
- Various drugs have been tried, with mixed results. Evidence currently only based on case studies. The following drugs have been tried:
  - amitriptyline;
  - gabapentin.[5]

Dysautonomia

Definition

Is a newly recognized condition in children where the autonomic nervous system appears to malfunction.

Symptoms

Include tachycardia, bradycardia, hypothermia, hyperthermia, pallor, flushing, retching, vomiting, bowel dysmotility, constipation, urinary retention, abnormal sweating, increased salivation, posturing, agitation, generalized discomfort, and abdominal pain.

Management
- Various drugs have been tried, with mixed results. Evidence currently only based on case studies. The following drugs have been tried:
  - benzodiazepine;
  - bromocriptine;
  - clonidine;
  - baclofen;
  - β antagonists;
  - morphine;
  - cyproheptadine;
  - gabapentin;
  - pregabalin.[5]

References

1. Nayak, S. and Cunliffe, M. (2008). Lidocaine 5% patch for localized chronic neuropathic pain in adolescents: report of five cases. *Paediatr. Anaesth.* **18** (6), 554–8.
2. Davies, D., DeVlaming, D., and Haines, C. (2008). Methadone analgesia for children with advanced cancer. *Pediatr. Blood Cancer* **51** (3), 393–7.
3. Colvin, L. and Fallon, M. (2008). Challenges in cancer pain management—bone pain. *Eur. J. Cancer* **44** (8), 1083–90.
4. Wagner, S., Poirot, I., Vuillerot, C., and Berard, C. (2011). Tolerance and effectiveness on pain control of Pamidronate® intravenous infusions in children with neuromuscular disorders. *Ann. Phys. Rehabil. Med.* **54** (6), 348–58.
5. Hauer, J.M. and Faulkner, K.W. (2012). Neurological and neuromuscular conditions and symptoms. In: Goldman, A., Hain, R., and Liben, S., editors. *Oxford textbook of palliative care for children*, second edition, pp. 295–300. Oxford University Press, Oxford.

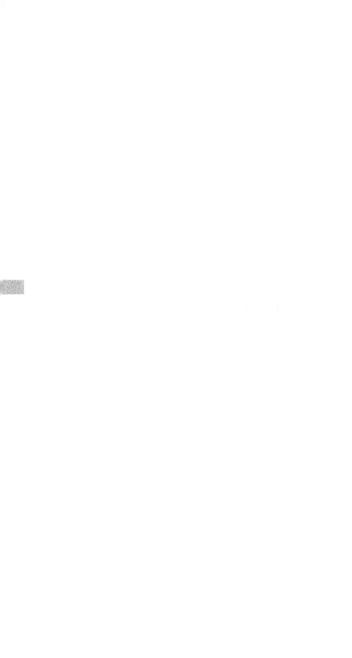

Nausea and vomiting

Introduction

The management of nausea and vomiting requires an understanding of the probable mechanism and a logical consideration of drug selection. But it also requires an approach that is individualized to the emotional and psychological needs of the child and family.

The evolutionary purpose of vomiting is to expel ingested toxins before they can do damage. Vomiting gives the body several opportunities to do this.

- Even the smell or sight of something nauseous can evoke a powerful emetic response (anticipatory nausea).
- Once a toxin is ingested, emesis can be initiated in the gastrointestinal tract, the liver, or the brain.
- It is mediated by a series of receptors and neurochemicals, modified (and often amplified) by emotional and psychological input from higher cortical centres, coordinated by a specialized centre of the brain, and finally effected via the vagus nerve.

Palliative medicine concerns patients in whom:

- anxiety levels are often high;
- there may be a multiplicity of physical factors.

Effective management of the symptom requires attention to all dimensions. This involves the following.

- It is important to explore the expectations of the patient and family before embarking on treatment.
- It is also important to be realistic about what can be achieved.
- Even with optimal pharmacological and psychological support, it is not always possible to abolish nausea and vomiting entirely.
- For most patients, reducing the frequency of vomiting to once or twice a day may be enough.
- As always, there is a need to balance the likely impact of antiemetic therapy against the potential adverse effects. The balance of burden and benefit for individual families needs to be established before embarking on treatment.

Pathophysiology: receptors

Most research in children has been in nausea and vomiting associated with chemotherapy.[1,2] Nausea and vomiting is known to be a significant symptom amongst children needing palliative care, particularly in cancer.[3–5] A rational approach in adults[6] has been proposed, but never validated in children.

The mechanism of the physiological basis of nausea and vomiting is essentially an interaction of neurochemicals with receptors. Each of the organs primarily involved in nausea and vomiting is associated with a group of receptors. Most antiemetics work by blocking one or more of the receptors. No antiemetic blocks all receptors.

Most is known about six antiemetic receptors.

- D_2 dopamine receptor. Found in the gastrointestinal tract and centrally. Blocked by metoclopramide and haloperidol.
- H_1 histamine receptor. Associated with intracranial and vestibular causes, blocked, along with acetylcholine (ACh), by cyclizine.
- ACh associated with vestibular causes and with the vagal nerve. Hyoscine is a pure ACh blocker.
- 5-hydroxytryptamine $(5HT)_2$ serotonin receptor. Associated with the bowel wall; blocked, amongst other things, by levomepromazine.
- $5HT_3$. Associated with the bowel wall; blocked by ondansetron and similar drugs.
- $5HT_4$. Associated with the bowel wall; blocked by high-dose metoclopramide.

A further class of receptors has recently been identified, with three subtypes associated with the bowel mucosa. They are neurokinin receptors NK_1, NK_2, and NK_3. This further opens up the possibilities for pharmacological intervention using antagonists. To date, only one neurokinin antagonist has been fully developed. Aprepitant, a pure NK_1 antagonist, has been studied in adults and appears to be well tolerated with good effect.[7]

Organs

Four organs are particularly involved in nausea and vomiting: the gastrointestinal tract; the bloodstream; the liver; and the brain. In considering a rational approach to managing nausea and vomiting, it is first necessary to decide which of these is or are the main cause(s).

Gastrointestinal

- Mucosal damage:
  - chemotherapy $(D_2, 5HT_3)$;
  - radiotherapy $(5HT_3, 5HT_4)$;
  - obstruction.
- Mechanical:
  - obstruction;
  - reflux.

Blood (toxins)

- Medication (D_2).
- Infection $(5HT_2)$.
- Constipation $(5HT_3, 5HT_4)$.

Liver damage
- Focal deposits (physical effect).
- Diffuse disease ($5HT_4$).

Brain
- Vestibular:
  - vertigo (ACh);
  - travel sickness (H_1).
- Raised intracranial pressure:
  - tumour (H_1);
  - oedema.
- Psychological:
  - anticipation;
  - anxiety (benzodiazepine receptors).

The motor pattern that constitutes the act of vomiting is generated in a specialized part of the brain, the vomiting centre (also known as the emetic pattern generator), and effected via the vagus nerve (ACh).

Pathophysiology: non-receptor mechanisms

Drug–receptor interactions are not the only links in the chain of causality for nausea and vomiting. It may be possible to modify other factors.

Physical factors

Can contribute to:

- raised intracranial pressure (e.g. brain tumour, cerebral oedema);
- liver damage (e.g. metastatic cancer, particularly where the liver capsule is stretched);
- gastrointestinal obstruction;
- reflux.

Psychological factors

There is often a close association between anxiety and nausea and vomiting. Two common situations are the following.

Anticipation

Commonly occurs when there is a strong association between an eme-togenic stimulus, such as chemotherapy, and a specific environment, such as oncology outpatients, in which sight, sound, and especially smell combine to reinforce the association over succeeding visits.

The association between environment, event, and emesis needs to be broken. This can be done using:

- play or psychotherapy;
- hypnotherapy;
- medications that attenuate the experience of anxiety, particularly nabilone (mildly euphoric derivative of marijuana with sedative and antiemetic properties) and benzodiazepines;
- complementary therapies.

Generalized anxiety

The above measures may be used. Benzodiazepines are anxiolytic, whereas soporifics (e.g. chloral hydrate, levomepromazine) are not.

- Midazolam. Can be given parenterally or buccally.
  - Advantage: rapid onset, short-acting, amnestic.
  - Disadvantages: may be so short-acting that it does not encompass the whole stressful episode.
- Lorazepam. May be given orally, parenterally, or sublingually.
  - Advantages: longer-acting, can be rapid-onset if given sublingually.
  - Disadvantages: long duration of action may not always be desirable.
- Diazepam. Can be given orally or parenterally or rectally.
  - Advantages: longer-acting.
  - Disadvantages: may be too long-acting.

In general, as with most medications for managing psychological aspects of illness, they should not be prescribed alone, but in association with appropriate non-drug techniques.

Management

Rational drug management of nausea and vomiting depends on:
- inferring or demonstrating what mechanisms are at work;
- understanding what receptors are likely to be involved;
- understanding what non-receptor mechanisms are likely to be involved.

Before embarking on medications

- Invasive investigations may not be justified in children close to death, as a diagnosis and rational management plan are usually possible without it.
- It is often not possible to abolish nausea and vomiting entirely, and this needs to be made clear from the outset, along with the assurance that significant improvement is very likely.
- Establish with the child and family what their goals are for managing the problem.
- Consider non-physical contributions to the symptom, and also physical contributions that can be managed in a non-pharmacological way (see ➲ Chapter 8, Pathophysiology: non-receptor mechanisms, p. 75).

Medications

Pharmacologically, a logical approach is as follows.
- Choose a rational first-line drug (i.e. one likely to block the appropriate receptors).
- Review the effectiveness of this approach.
- If this fails, choose a rational second-line drug. This can be one of three things:
  - an alternative drug, because, in the meantime, an alternative explanation for the problem has become clear;
  - a complementary drug, i.e. one that blocks some of the receptors that were not blocked by your first choice;
  - an alternative antiemetic that blocks a much wider range of receptors. Phenothiazines, and in particular levomepromazine, are 'broad-spectrum' antiemetics and can be useful second-line drugs.

Table 8.1 shows the receptor antagonist properties of common antiemetics. On the basis of an understanding of those receptor properties and of the likely mechanism of nausea and vomiting in your patient, it should be possible to derive a logical approach.

Steroids

Long-term steroids should be avoided in PPM, as their benefits are quickly outweighed by their adverse effects. Short courses of steroids may, however, be helpful adjuvants in managing nausea and vomiting. Steroids probably do not work directly through a drug–receptor interaction, but by:
- reducing oedema, particularly in the brain (e.g. brain tumour) or in the liver (e.g. infection or metastatic disease);
- reducing inflammation; by moderating the inflammatory response, steroids can reduce the amount of cell damage and release of mediators of emesis.

Table 8.1 Some causes of nausea and vomiting and appropriate antiemetics for treating them

Likely cause	Example	Antiemetic (receptor)
Vestibular	Vertigo or travel sickness	Hyoscine (ACh) or cyclizine (ACh, H_1)
Toxins	Medications, particularly chemotherapy Infections (endotoxins) Constipation	Metoclopramide, haloperidol (D_2) Ondansetron, etc. ($5HT_3$) Metoclopramide ($5HT_4$)
Gastrointestinal damage	Chemotherapy	Metoclopramide (D_2, $5HT_4$) Ondansetron, etc. ($5HT_3$) Steroids (inflammation)
Liver damage	Focal deposits Diffuse disease	Metoclopramide ($5HT_4$) Steroids (inflammation)
Psychological	Anticipation and anxiety	Non-physical Benzodiazepine receptors Nabilone
Raised intracranial pressure	Tumour Oedema	Cyclizine (H_1) Steroids (oedema)

Metoclopramide and domperidone

The European Medicines Agency (EMA) recommended a change to the use of metoclopramide[8] (2013) and domperidone[9] (2014) to restrict the dose and duration, to minimize known risks of potential neurological and cardiac side effects. The restriction does not apply to palliative care, as the guidance only covers licensed indications. As such, prescribers in PPM are advised to be fully knowledgeable of the guidance and encompass this information during their discussion with the patient or family when recommending the use these drugs in an unlicensed way. However, they are not limited in terms of dosage or duration by the new guidance, and one should prescribe what is best for the child.

Reflux

In children with life-limiting conditions that are non-malignant, reflux is an important differential diagnosis from true nausea and vomiting. The main causes are:

- a lax gastro-oesophageal sphincter caused by muscle incoordination;
- painful and dangerous acid reflux;
- loss of normal reflex bowel motility, causing overdistension, particularly by continuous feeds.

Each of these factors can be managed rationally.
- Lax gastro-oesophageal sphincter:
  - D_2 blockers, e.g. metoclopramide.
- Painful and dangerous acid reflux:
  - H_2 blockers, e.g. ranitidine;
  - proton blockers, e.g. omeprazole;
  - alginates, e.g. Gaviscon®.
- Loss of normal reflex bowel motility:
  - change feed timings to avoid an overfull stomach;
  - dopamine blockers.

Rational approach to antiemesis

Box 8.1 and Fig. 8.1 summarize a rational approach to the treatment of nausea and vomiting.

Box 8.1 Summary of antiemetic approaches

- All children:
  - explain, reassure, and modify the diet, to ensure it consists of frequent, low-volume, attractive foods;
  - treat anxiety (see ➲ Chapter 13).
- Possible iatrogenic causes?
  - review the drug list, and stop non-essential emetogenic drugs.
- Non-pharmacological management?
  - anxiety reduction (see ➲ Chapter 13).
- Features of gastritis or oesophagitis (pain, indigestion, flatulence, blood in vomit)?
  - stop NSAIDs and steroids, if possible;
  - use omeprazole or ranitidine;
  - add alginate.
- Features of gastric stasis or compression (e.g. known abdominal tumour or abdominal organomegaly)?
  - try gastric motility stimulant (domperidone or metoclopramide).
- Related to movement?
  - rule out an iatrogenic cause;
  - start a vestibular-active drug such as cyclizine or hyoscine hydrobromide.
- Related to toxic or systemic causes (e.g. infections, advanced tumours, renal or hepatic failure)?
  - treat the underlying cause where possible;
  - use drugs active on central nervous system (CNS) receptors such as promazine, haloperidol, cyclizine.
- Features of raised intracranial pressure?
  - consider radiotherapy or a shunt;
  - if not appropriate, cyclizine is the drug of choice;
  - consider steroids, but see cautions in Chapter 12.
- Above suggestions not working, or is sedation indicated?
  - try levomepromazine (if available).

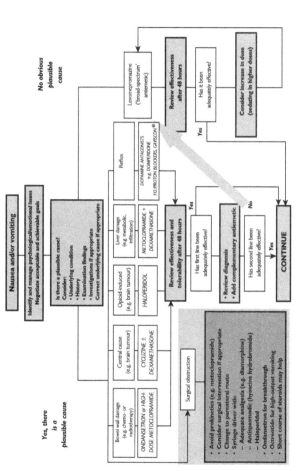

Fig. 8.1 A flow chart outlining a rational approach to antemesis.

Summary of nausea and vomiting

- Evaluate, negotiate, and investigate only as appropriate for the individual child in the individual family.
- Choose a rational first-line drug, based on an understanding of the likely aetiology and of antiemetic pharmacology.
- Review effectiveness and tolerability.
- If ineffective, choose a rational alternative or complement, or switch to a broad-spectrum antiemetic, such as levomepromazine, which blocks many receptors.
- Always consider psychosocial and emotional components, and address these using non-drug and drug interventions.

References

1. Antonarakis, E.S., Evans, J.L., Heard, G.F., Noonan, L.M., Pizer, L., and Hain, R. (2004). Prophylaxis of acute chemotherapy-induced nausea and vomiting in children with cancer: what is the evidence? *Pediatr. Blood Cancer* **43** (6), 651–8.
2. Antonarakis, E.S. and Hain, R. (2004). Nausea and vomiting associated with cancer chemotherapy: drug management in theory and in practice. *Arch. Dis. Child* **89** (9), 877–80.
3. Goldman, A., Hewitt, M., Collins, G.S., Childs, M., and Hain, R. (2006). Symptoms in children/young people with progressive malignant disease: United Kingdom Children's Cancer Study Group/Paediatric Oncology Nurses Forum survey. *Pediatrics* **117** (6), e1179–86.
4. Hongo, T., Watanabe, C., Okada, S., Inoue, N., Yajima, S., Fujii, Y., et al. (2003). Analysis of the circumstances at the end of life in children with cancer: symptoms, suffering and acceptance. *Pediatr. Int.* **45** (1), 60–4.
5. Wolfe, J., Grier, H.E., Klar, N., Levin, S.B., Ellenbogen, J.M., Salem-Schatz, S., et al. (2000). Symptoms and suffering at the end of life in children with cancer [see comments]. *N. Engl. J. Med.* **342** (5), 326–33.
6. Twycross, R. and Back, I. (1998). Nausea and vomiting in advanced cancer. *Eur. J. Palliative Care* **5** (2), 39–45.
7. Warr, D.G., Hesketh, P.J., Gralla, R.J., Muss, H.B., Herrstedt, J., Eisenberg, P.D., et al. (2005). Efficacy and tolerability of aprepitant for the prevention of chemotherapy-induced nausea and vomiting in patients with breast cancer after moderately emetogenic chemotherapy. *J. Clin. Oncol.* **23** (12), 2822–30.
8. European Medicines Agency (2013). *European Medicines Agency recommends changes to the use of metoclopramide.* Available at: ℘ http://www.ema.europa.eu/docs/en_GB/document_library/Press_release/2013/07/WC500146614.pdf.
9. European Medicines Agency (2014). *Restrictions on the use of domperidone-containing medicines.* Available at: ℘ http://www.ema.europa.eu/docs/en_GB/document_library/Referrals_document/Domperidone_31/European_Commission_final_decision/WC500172573.pdf.

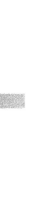

Chapter 9

Gastrointestinal symptoms

Constipation

Definition

- Normal frequency is variable and age-dependent:
  - breastfed baby—once or twice a week, up to ten times a day;
  - toddlers—twice a day;
  - older—three times a day to three times a week.
- Constipation represents a reduction in bowel frequency from normal for the child that causes symptoms.

General points

- Structured formal assessment (including medical, drug, dietary, and social history and appropriate examination) may establish a cause and permit rational choice of intervention. This requires good communication with carers and often uncovers misconceptions about 'normal' defecation and the use of laxatives.
- Rectal examination is distressing and should be avoided, if possible, especially after repeated examinations or in the presence of an anal tear. If unavoidable, it should be done by an experienced professional after appropriate discussion.
- Severe constipation can masquerade as faecal soiling or frank diarrhoea as a result of impaction and overflow.

Management of constipation

Causes

- Inactivity due to illness or treatment (e.g. chemotherapy, physical and/or cognitive impairment).
- Dehydration.
- Abnormal feeding patterns and/or reduced intake.
- Specific effects of an illness: cystic fibrosis, hypercalcaemia, or hypokalaemia.
- Psychosocial: loss of dignity, lack of privacy, unfamiliar toilets, reluctance to alert carers to a need to defecate.
- Anal tears (often from passing hard stools).
- Drugs, including many used in palliative care, especially opioids, anticholinergics, and $5HT_3$.

Treatment

- If possible, reverse the cause (e.g. dehydration). Dietary manipulation can be important but is often complicated by chewing and swallowing difficulties.
- Choose a rational laxative (see ➔ Chapter 26):
  - *stimulant* if reduced motility seems likely;
  - *softener* if hard stool is present (often together with the above);
  - *oral naloxone* if opioid-induced;
  - *combination of softeners and 48-hourly glycerin suppositories* in paraplegia);
  - *topical anaesthetic gel*, e.g. lidocaine ointment (or even a short general anaesthetic) if anal fissure apparent or manual removal is required.

- If no rational approach is possible, use paediatric Movicol®.
- If that is ineffective, a pragmatic plan is:
  - step 1. Osmotic laxative, building up the dose slowly over a week;
  - step 2. If no improvement, add a stimulant laxative, such as senna, or change to co-danthramer (only licensed in palliative care);
  - step 3. If constipation persists, then perform a rectal examination:
    — if stool hard, use a lubricant suppository such as glycerin;
    — if stool soft, use a stimulant suppository such as bisacodyl;
    — if rectum empty, use a bisacodyl suppository to bring the stool down, or a high-phosphate enema.
  - step 4. If severely constipated, use Micralax® or a phosphate enema.

Novel approaches
- Oral naloxone has been used in adult care to alleviate opioid-induced constipation.
- Erythromycin has a side effect of increased bowel motility, and this has been used successfully in resistant cases.
- Prokinetic drugs, such as metoclopramide or domperidone, have all been tried, with varying success.

Diarrhoea

Causes
- Severe constipation can masquerade as faecal soiling or frank diarrhoea as a result of impaction and overflow.
- Gastroenteritis.
- HIV/AIDS most common palliative cause in the world.
- Faecal impaction.
- Malabsorption/diet.
- Pancreatic exocrine deficiency (cystic fibrosis).
- Drug-induced:
  - directly (e.g. NSAID);
  - indirectly (e.g. antibiotics).
- Post-radiation/chemotherapy.
- Concurrent illness such as colitis.

Management
- Fluid management:
  - clear fluids;
  - electrolyte replacement;
  - parenteral fluids (using hypodermoclysis if iv access not readily available).
- Correction of reversible causes.
- Live yoghurt.
- Specific antimicrobial, fungicidal, and antiparasitic treatment, particularly in HIV-related diarrhoea.
- Pancreatic enzyme replacement.
- Empiric drug treatment (e.g. morphine, loperamide, co-phenotrope).
- For severe high-output diarrhoea in palliative care, consider a long-acting somatostatin analogue (octreotide):
  - increases fluid absorption from the bowel;
  - improves peristalsis;
  - only available parenterally (sc infusion or intermittent injection);
  - effects can be dramatic but short-lived.

Sialorrhoea

Definition
Difficulty in swallowing saliva or (less commonly) over-production of saliva, leading to persistent 'drooling' from the mouth.

Physiology
Sialorrhoea can be caused by three different factors:
- excessive production of saliva;
- inability to retain saliva in the mouth;
- difficulty in swallowing.

Excessive production is not a problem in itself, unless accompanied by one or both of the other two factors.

Symptoms
- Dermatitis around the mouth, lips, and chin.
- Constant need to change bibs and clothing.
- Choking.
- Coughing.
- Aspiration pneumonia.
- Dysphagia.
- Breathing difficulties.
- Social stigma.

Causes
- Neurodegenerative disorders: 10% of all cases, and up to half of all children with cerebral palsy.
- Abnormalities of the mouth, jaw, or nasopharynx.
- Cancer affecting the mouth.
- Dysphagia.
- Psychological.
- Drugs (e.g. cholinergic drugs, neuroleptics).

Management
Saliva consists of two components, a thin watery secretion and a thick mucus. These are produced by different salivary glands. Treatment tends to affect these two components differently and can cause the paradoxical problem of reducing saliva production but producing thick mucus in the throat that is difficult to cough up.

Treatment requires a logical and pragmatic approach. Pharmacological treatments only work in 50% of cases and, even then, become less effective over time.
- Treat local factors:
    - dental hygiene;
    - dermatitis with mild steroids, antibiotics, moisturizers, or barrier creams;
    - sore gums and mouth ulcers with topical analgesics.
- Review medication, which may be exacerbating the problem.

Scopolamine (hyoscine hydrobromide)
- Comes in various formulations, but patch most useful, as it avoids first-pass liver effect, so smaller doses can be used.
- Lasts 72h, so not suitable for sialorrhoea that is variable.
- Smaller doses can be given by occluding part of the patch. In our unit, we cut the patch, although this is out of licence.
- Side effects include: behavioural problems, constipation, cardiac arrhythmia, urinary retention, flushing, nausea, giddiness and confusion, restlessness, and blurred vision.
- Has been given sublingually or as drops.[1]

Glycopyrronium bromide
- Suitable for sialorrhoea that is variable.
- Available in oral formulation.
- Similar effectiveness, and side effects to hyoscine.
- Tends to cause fewer central effects such as confusion.

Botulinum toxin A
- Injected into the parotid and submandibular glands.
- Should be done under ultrasound control, as injection into other sites may lead to paralysis of critical muscles.
- Evidence in adults suggests good and sustained effectiveness in severe sialorrhoea.[2]

Surgery
- Outcome often poor.
- Three possible approaches:
  - removing salivary glands;
  - ligating salivary ducts;
  - sectioning the nerve supply (denervation procedures reduce taste to the anterior two-thirds of the tongue).
- Current recommendation is ligation of the parotid and submandibular glands.

Visceral hyperalgesia

Definition

Severe, often intermittent, pain that has (or seems to have) an abdominal focus but which is not obviously caused by any demonstrable abnormality. It is a form of neuropathic pain.

- Hyperalgesia in older children, as a result of repeated noxious stimuli in the neonatal phase, is well recognized.
- There are sensory nerves in the bowel.
- Amongst children with life-limiting conditions (especially RCPCH/ACT categories 2, 3, and 4), repeated damage to the bowel is common (e.g. necrotizing enterocolitis, hypoxia, feeding).
- Those noxious stimuli may cause a form of hyperalgesia in the bowel and account for some severe abdominal pain in later life.
- There is no specific diagnostic test, but visceral hyperalgesia is strongly suggested by response to appropriate anti-neuropathic adjuvants.

Anorexia

Definition
Many different life-limiting conditions can reduce a child's desire to eat. Loss of appetite can cause considerable distress to the child's family, as feeding one's child is a deeply embedded and primal evolutionary instinct.

Causes
- Physical discomfort:
  - pain: either generalized or specific to eating (e.g. dyspepsia);
  - nausea, vomiting, or constipation;
  - difficulty swallowing (dysphagia), e.g. as a result of disease process;
  - thrush in the mouth or oesophagus;
  - xerostomia (e.g. from anticholinergics or radiotherapy).
- Loss of food appeal:
  - altered sense of taste or smell as a result of drugs, especially chemotherapy agents;
  - unappetizing presentation (e.g. hospital food);
  - psychological (e.g. anxiety, depression).

Management
At the end of life, anorexia is normal, and any decision to intervene should be taken cautiously. There is a risk of prescribing medications to a child, in order to treat their parents' need to feed them.
- Reassure parents that an inactive child will have a reduced requirement for food.
- Treat reversible causes, especially pain.
- Make food more appealing:
  - use smaller portions;
  - use smaller plates;
  - encourage more frequent meals;
  - allow parents to give favourite foods (e.g. McDonald's);
  - be flexible with timings of meals;
  - make food that require less effort to eat—mash, soups, etc.
- Food supplements are unpleasant and may not be appropriate. They can be made less unpalatable by serving them cold. Involve a dietitian early if considering this approach.
- Anabolic steroids, such as prednisolone or dexamethasone, can be used in short 5- to 7-day bursts to increase appetite. Side effects, particularly those of body distortion, severely limit their longer-term use.
- Other medical stimulants of appetite include some antipsychotics and other psychoactive medications. Again, the potential adverse effects of these are significant, and they should be used with great caution in children.

Cachexia

Definition
A metabolic state of increased catabolism of fat and lean body mass, associated with a range of chemical mediators and leading to damage to skeletal muscle (particularly pale fibres). The result of cachexia is profound weight loss, lethargy, and fatigue. The resulting alteration of body image can be distressing to the child and family.

Causes
- Endogenous acute response to illness or injury.
- Linked with many chronic and end-stage conditions, but particularly cancer.
- More common in solid tumour cancers than in haematological cancers.
- Relatively rare in children, compared with adults.

Management
- Cachexia is not caused by low calorie intake. Unless it is associated with anorexia (see ➲ Chapter 9, Anorexia, p. 90), there is no benefit in using high-calorie diets.
- Several drug interventions are being tried in adults, but evidence of use in paediatrics is poor:
  - anabolic steroids;
  - human growth hormone;
  - testosterone;
  - appetite stimulants: megestrol;
  - NSAIDs;
  - cytokine antagonists;
  - nutritional supplements: omega-3 fatty acids.

Hiccough

Definition

Hiccough (or 'hiccup') describes an involuntary contraction of the diaphragm, resulting in sudden inspiration, followed by abrupt closure of the glottis. It is rare in the palliative care setting but, where it occurs, may have a pathological cause and need treatment, because it is distressing, persistent (i.e. lasting longer than 2 days), or intractable (lasting longer than 1 month).

Causes

- Gastrointestinal:
  - gastro-oesophageal reflux disease (GORD);
  - gastric distension;
  - diaphragmatic irritation.
- Phrenic nerve irritation.
- Biochemical:
  - uraemia;
  - hyponatraemia;
  - hypocalcaemia;
  - liver dysfunction.
- Stress and insomnia.
- Pyrexia.
- Infection.
- Intracranial lesion.
- Drugs:
  - corticosteroids;
  - antidepressants;
  - antibiotics;
  - analgesics, including opioids.
- Many of the drugs used to treat hiccoughs can also induce them.

Management

- Gastric distension:
  - defoaming antiflatulent such as Asilone® or Maalox® Plus;
  - prokinetic drug that tightens the lower oesophageal sphincter such as metoclopramide;
  - peppermint water relaxes the lower oesophageal sphincter to aid belching (do not use with metoclopramide).
- Management of gastro-oesophageal reflux (see ➔ Chapter 8):
  - metoclopramide;
  - H_2 antagonists;
  - proton pump inhibitors (PPIs).
- Diaphragmatic irritation:
  - baclofen as a muscle relaxant;
  - chlorpromazine;
  - reports in adults of benefits with nifedipine and midazolam.

- Vagal stimulation techniques:
  - normal saline, 2mL nebulized over 5min;
  - oropharyngeal stimulation with a nasogastric (NG) tube;
  - massage at the junction of the hard and soft palate with cotton bud;
  - forced retraction of the tongue to induce a gag reflex;
  - vagal stimulation through carotid massage or the Valsalva manoeuvre;
  - some folk remedies (e.g. swallowing crushed ice, cold key down the back, shouting 'boo' to produce a startle response).
- Central suppression of hiccough reflex:
  - metoclopramide;
  - chlorpromazine;
  - baclofen;
  - sodium valproate, phenytoin, or carbamazepine;
  - elevating $PaCO_2$ in the brainstem by breath-holding or breathing in and out of a paper bag.

Blended feeds

Feeds given via an enteral tube have traditionally been prepared under sterile and standardized conditions by pharmaceutical companies. Many parents are reluctant to use those prepared commercial products, preferring instead to blend feeds themselves, according to recipes. There are several reasons.

- They feel it is more 'normal' and less medicalized.
- Preparing food for one's child is a primal drive and an important part of family life.
- There is anecdotal evidence that it results in better bowel habit, perhaps by leading to a more normal population of the gut flora.
- It is less expensive in countries that lack a socialized health system such as the US.

In the UK, pharmaceutical companies and dietitians have been reluctant to endorse a move to feeds blended at home, because:

- they are not sterile;
- there is a risk of inadequate homogenization that might cause damage to equipment;
- they make it more difficult to control a child's calorie intake.

There is, however, little evidence to support the claim of high risk with home-prepared feeds, and objectors note that:

- the bowel is not normally a sterile environment, and most children receiving enteral feeds have no immune deficit that might make sterility important;
- the manufacturers of equipment are also the manufacturers of prescribed feeds, so there is a relevant conflict of interests. Their appropriate response should be to improve the equipment design, to minimize the risk of damage;
- for children with life-limiting conditions, close control of calorie intake is typically unnecessary.

In the absence of persuasive evidence of harm, there is little justification for preventing parents from choosing to feed their child in this manner. There are ongoing trials examining the safety and effectiveness of home-prepared blended feeds and ways in which they can be optimized.

References

1. Rapoport, A. (2010). Sublingual atropine drops for the treatment of pediatric sialorrhea. *J. Pain Symptom Manage.* **40** (5), 783–8.
2. Barbero, P., Busso, M., Tinivella, M., Artusi, C.A., De Mercanti, S., Cucci, A., *et al.* (2015). Long-term follow-up of ultrasound-guided botulinum toxin-A injections for sialorrhea in neurological dysphagia. *J. Neurol.* **262** (12), 2662–7.

Further reading

Bellomo-Brandao, M.A., Collares, E.F., and da-Costa-Pinto, E.A. (2003). Use of erythromycin for the treatment of severe chronic constipation in children. *Braz. J. Med. Biol. Res.* **36** (10), 1391–6.
British Dietetic Association (2015). *Policy statement: use of liquidised food with enteral feeding tubes.* British Dietetic Association, Birmingham. Available at: ℗ https://www.bda.uk.com/improving-health/healthprofessionals/policystatement_liquidisedfood.
Friedman, N.L. (1996). Hiccoughs: a treatment review. *Pharmacotherapy* **16** (6), 986–95.
Greensmith, A.L., Johnstone, B.R., Reid, S.M., Hazard, C.J., Johnson, H.M., and Reddihough, D.S. (2005). Prospective analysis of the outcome of surgical management of drooling in the pediatric population: a 10-year experience. *Plast. Reconstr. Surg.* **116** (5), 1233–42.
Meningaud, J.P., Pitak-Arnnop, P., Chikhani, L., and Bertrand, J.C. (2006). Drooling of saliva: a review of the etiology and management options. *Oral Surg. Oral Med. Oral Pathol. Oral Radiol. Endod.* **101** (1), 48–57.
Mercadante S. (1994). The role of octreotide in palliative care. *J. Pain Symptom Manage.* **9** (6), 406–11.
Miller, M. and Karwacki, M. (2012). Management of the gastrointestinal tract in paediatric palliative medicine. In: Goldman, A., Hain, R., and Liben, S., editors. *Oxford textbook of palliative care for children*, second edition, pp. 271–83. Oxford University Press, Oxford.
Miranda, A. (2008). Early life events and the development of visceral hyperalgesia. *J. Pediatr. Gastroenterol. Nutr.* **47** (5), 682–4.
Tofil, N.M., Benner, K.W., Faro, S.J., and Winkler, M.K. (2006). The use of enteral naloxone to treat opioid-induced constipation in a pediatric intensive care unit. *Pediatr. Crit. Care Med.* **7** (3), 252–4.

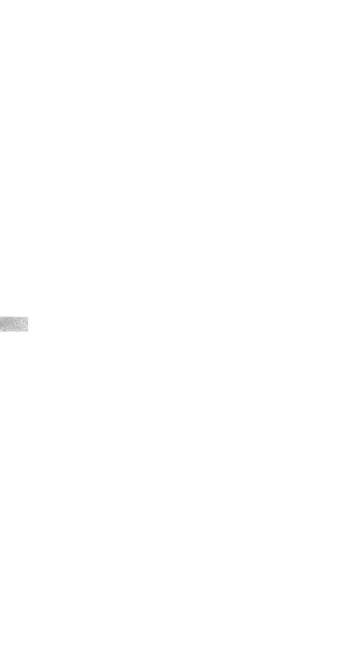

Mouth care, feeding, and hydration

Mouth care

General points

- This is an often overlooked area of symptom management, as doctors typically have little training in oral medicine.
- Pathology in the mouth can have a considerable effect on the child's ability to communicate and to eat.
- Maintenance of oral hygiene can often be done by parents, and this allows them to be actively involved in helping their child through actions that are perceived to be part of normal parenting.
- Successful management can considerably improve the quality of a child's life.
- Be aware that a high-sugar diet (including medication) can lead to tooth decay.
- Correct management requires taking a good history, always looking inside the mouth, and basic clinical skills.

Cause of mouth symptoms

- Poor oral hygiene.
- Oral candidiasis:
  - antibiotics;
  - corticosteroids;
  - general debility.
- Dry mouth:
  - mouth breathing;
  - dehydration;
  - oxygen that has not been humidified;
  - anxiety;
  - drugs: opioids, antihistamines, antimuscarinics, antidepressants, diuretics;
  - radiotherapy;
  - stomatitis secondary to neutropenia;
  - direct damage to salivary glands from tumour infiltration or radiotherapy;
  - hypercalcaemia or hyperglycaemia.
- Mouth ulcers:
  - infection;
  - traumatic;
  - aphthous.
- Bleeding gums:
  - poor oral hygiene;
  - haematological cancers;
  - liver disease;
  - clotting disorders.

Management

- Poor oral hygiene.
  - Pink sponges or gauze dipped in mouthwash or water, applied to gums and teeth.
  - Clean a furred tongue with a soft toothbrush or with effervescent mouthwash tablets (vitamin C).
  - Use pineapple chunks sucked as sweets to clean the mouth (contains an enzyme ananase).
  - Antiseptic mouthwashes or gel, e.g. chlorhexidine.
  - Refer to a dentist or hygienist for removal of hard plaque deposits and oral hygiene instruction.
- Oral candidiasis.[1]
  - Nystatin works as a topical agent, but not always successful in children due to difficulty getting them to retain the solution in the mouth.
  - Miconazole gel retains well in the mouth; has both local and systemic effects.
  - Fluconazole: once-daily oral agent, with high success rate.
- Dry mouth.[2]
  - Correct dehydration.
  - Use a humidifier with oxygen.
  - Reassess all medications, and rationalize.
  - Apply petroleum jelly, e.g. Vaseline™ or K-Y™ jelly, to lips.
  - Stimulate salivation with ice chips, chewing gum, or citrus sweets and drinks.
  - Use artificial saliva such as Glandosane®.
  - Parasympathomimetics have been used in adult palliative care, but there is no experience in children.
- Mouth ulcers.
  - Assessment by a dentist.
  - Antiseptic mouthwashes: chlorhexidine.
  - Corticosteroids for aphthous ulcers: triamcinolone or hydrocortisone lozenges.
- Bleeding gums.
  - Improve oral hygiene.
  - Tranexamic acid mouthwashes.
  - Haemostatic agents: Gelfoam® or Gelfilm®.
  - Platelet transfusion may be required in some haematological disorders/malignancies.

Feeding

General points

- Feeding one's child is a basic parental instinct, so a situation where this is causing problems is very distressing not only for the child, but also the family.
- Loss of appetite and weight loss occur in many advanced cancers.
- Children with neurological problems experience a lot of difficulties with feeding, including: prolonged feeding time, choking, vomiting, constipation, recurrent chest infections, and poor weight gain.[3]
- Artificial feeding carries many benefits but may also be a burden.
- Artificial feeding is not always perceived by parents as a positive experience.
- The general principles behind the ethics of feeding are discussed in Chapter 3.
- Management of feeding problems should begin with a diagnosis.
- Management of feeding requires a multidisciplinary approach, with the major lead coming from dietitians.[4]

Nutritional assessment

- Assessment of the clinical condition, its state of progression, and the effect of all the different stages on feeding and nutrition.
- Feeding history.
- Social assessment.
- Ability to chew, swallow, and digest.
- Medication review, looking for drugs that affect appetite or taste and drugs that alter absorption of nutrients.
- Serial weight and height measurements.
- Selected laboratory tests.
- Assessment of the nutritional requirement of a child should be based on the above and any specific nutritional effects or requirements of their condition.

Factors that may help when feeding

- Position.
- Seating.
- Feeding equipment.
- Person doing the feeding to be relaxed and calm.
- Positive reinforcement.
- Distraction techniques.
- Accept that feeding may be a lengthy process or time-consuming.
- Alter food:
  - use smaller portions;
  - use smaller plates;
  - encourage more frequent meals;
  - allow parents to give their children 'fast foods';
  - be flexible with timings of meals;
  - make food less effort to eat—mash, soups, etc.

- Involve a dietitian early.
- If the child experiences abnormal taste:
  - metallic tastes from chemotherapy can be reduced by tart foods such as lemon juice, pickles, etc.;
  - foods with their own flavours such as fruit and boiled sweets;
  - reduce the urea content of diet with specific food.
- Add calorie-rich food to meals, e.g. cheese, cream, etc.
- Energy and nutritional supplements.
- Treat reflux, dyspepsia, constipation, etc.

Enteral feeding

Factors that would influence the need for enteral feeding

- Significant risk of aspiration.
- Poor weight gain or weight loss.
- Weight below the second percentile.
- Child unable to swallow food or medication.
- More than 4h a day spent on feeding.
- Significant risk of dehydration due to poor swallowing.
- Where the benefits of enteral feeding outweigh the burdens.
- Modifications to feeding regimens can provide a solution to some symptoms such as reflux vomiting. This should ideally always be in collaboration with a dietitian.[5]

Nasogastric tube

Benefits

- Cheap.
- Easy to insert—can be done by parents after suitable training.
- Fine-bore tube now available.
- Polyurethane tubes can be left in 4–6 weeks, before needing changing.
- Does not require hospital admission or general anaesthetic.

Problems

- Body image.
- Can be traumatic to insert.
- Misplacement in the lungs or small intestine.
- Nasal/skin irritation.
- Can be pulled out easily by young children.
- Accidental removal.
- Easily occluded.
- Only medications in a suitable form can be passed down the tube.

Gastrostomy

Benefits

- Ideal choice for children requiring feeding for more than 3 months.
- Socially more acceptable.
- Less likely to be taken out or fall out.
- Can be used for overnight feeding.
- Management is easy for parents.
- Experience of fitting now developed by many paediatric surgeons, with excellent results.

Problems

- Occlusion.
- Granulation tissue formation.
- Requires general anaesthetic to fit (new technique of using radiologically inserted gastrostomy without general anaesthetic in adults has now started being used in teenagers).
- Infection.
- Tube can fall or be pulled out.
- Body image.
- If gastro-oesophageal reflux present, then may require fundoplication.[6]
- Only medications in a suitable form can be passed down the tube.

Gastrostomy blockage

In the event of a blockage, the following can be tried.[7] Using a 50mL syringe (smaller syringes can create too great a pressure and damage the tube), the following fluids (25–30mL) can be used (as age-appropriate) to unblock the tube, usually a minimum of 10mL.

- Flush with warm water.
- Flush with soda water.
- Flush with cola or pineapple juice.
- Try gently drawing back on the syringe.
- Squeeze along the length (milking) of the tube.
- For a percutaneous endoscopic gastrostomy (PEG), use pancreatic enzyme (Pancrex V®); instil, and leave for 30min.
- For Mic-Key, consider changing the tube.

Blended feeds

Feeds given down a tube have traditionally been manufactured products prescribed by the health-care team. Increasingly, many parents are choosing to use feeds they have prepared themselves. Although it is the right of parents to feed their child in any way that will be effective and safe, the practice is controversial, because there are hypothetical risks, as well as benefits.

Risks

- More difficult to monitor and ensure adequate calorie intake (though this may not be as significant for children in later stages of life-limiting conditions).
- Greater risk that parents will adopt idiosyncratic diets that are, in fact, harmful to the child.
- Home-prepared feeds are not aseptic, so greater risk of infection (though this is also true of normal food and may only be relevant to children with particular vulnerability to infection).
- Companies that manufacture feeds design tubes with those feeds in mind. Home-prepared feeds are less homogenous than manufactured products, and there is a greater risk of damage to equipment, particularly the tubes themselves (though, properly considered, that is a flaw in the design of the equipment which the manufacturers should address).

Benefits

Parents report various benefits, especially:

- emotional benefit to the family of being able to nourish one's own child;
- social benefit to the child of being able to share the same food as the rest of the family;
- more normal stools and bowel activity, perhaps as a result of normalizing the gut flora;
- less abdominal pain;
- less expensive. Important in resource-poor countries or where the cost of manufactured feeds is not covered by socialized health care.

The recommendations of professional bodies have often been cautious,[8] but, at the time of writing, none of the claims of significant harm is unequivocally supported by available evidence. Until such evidence emerges, it seems unreasonable for those working in palliative care not to help parents who wish to prepare their own feeds to do so appropriately.

Hydration

General points

- Hydration in the palliative care setting is normally via the oral or enteral route.
- Isotonic fluids can be usually given via the sc route, if necessary.
- Children in the terminal phase of their illness can often be left mildly fluid-restricted to reduce terminal secretion.
- The younger the child, the less well they tolerate variations of fluid balance.
- Fluid balance is based on weight, and not age.
- The calculation is based on advanced paediatric life support (APLS) recommendations.[9]

References

1. Lavy, V. (2007). Presenting symptoms and signs in children referred for palliative care in Malawi. *Palliat. Med.* **21** (4), 333–9.
2. Duval, M. and Wood, C. (2002). [Treatment of non-painful symptoms in terminally ill children]. *Arch. Pediatr.* **9** (11), 1173–8.
3. Sullivan, P.B., Lambert, B., Rose, M., Ford-Adams, M., Griffiths, P., and Johnson, A. (2000). Prevalence and severity of feeding and nutritional problems in children with neurological impairment: Oxford Feeding Study. *Dev. Med. Child Neurol.* **42** (10), 674–80.
4. Ayoob, K.T. and Barresi, I. (2007). Feeding disorders in children: taking an interdisciplinary approach. *Pediatr. Ann.* **36** (8), 478–83.
5. Motion, S., Northstone, K., Emond, A., Stucke, S., and Golding, J. (2002). Early feeding problems in children with cerebral palsy: weight and neurodevelopmental outcomes. *Dev. Med. Child Neurol.* **44** (1), 40–3.
6. Samuel, M. and Holmes, K. (2002). Quantitative and qualitative analysis of gastroesophageal reflux after percutaneous endoscopic gastrostomy. *J. Pediatr. Surg.* **37** (2), 256–61.
7. Jassal, S. (2007). *Basic symptom control in paediatric palliative care, the Rainbows Children's Hospice guidelines*, seventh edition. Rainbows Children's Hospice, Loughborough.
8. British Dietetic Association (2015). *Policy statement: use of liquidised food with enteral feeding tubes.* British Dietetic Association, Birmingham. Available at: ℅ https://www.bda.uk.com/improving-health/healthprofessionals/policystatement_liquidisedfood.
9. Advanced Life Support Group (2005). *Advanced paediatric life support*, fourth edition. BMJ Books, London.

Dyspnoea

Introduction

The principles that underlie the management of dyspnoea are the same as those underlying the management of any other symptom, namely:

- holistic;
- rational;
- balancing burden and benefit.

Holistic approach

Dyspnoea is defined as the sense that breathing has become unpleasant. It is therefore, by definition, a subjective phenomenon. It also means that many different factors can contribute to dyspnoea. These include:

- physical factors (fluid, tumour, weakness, injury);
- psychosocial factors (fears about function, inability to carry out normal tasks such as walking or feeding);
- existential or spiritual (interference with respiratory function carries implication of imminent death, fear of suffocation).

Dyspnoea is subjective

It is important to remember that there is only limited correlation between the observation of disordered breathing (e.g. tachypnoea) and the experience of dyspnoea. Breathing can be unpleasant without being abnormal, and can be abnormal without being unpleasant.

The multidimensional significance of difficulty in breathing is highlighted by the dual meanings of the terms 'inspire' and 'expire'. The word 'spirit' itself is related both to breath and to the essence of life. The sensation that breathing has ceased to be effortless and has become unpleasant or difficult carries with it emotional weight that goes well beyond the physical. Conversely, breathing that is abnormal to an observer without being unpleasant. An obvious example is the tachypnoea associated with ketoacidosis.

Pathophysiology

It is helpful to consider the possible causes for dyspnoea by considering, in turn, all the parts of the respiratory system from the diaphragm to the respiratory centre.

Muscle weakness
- Causes:
  - cachexia;
  - DMD;
  - other neuromuscular degenerative conditions.
- Interventions:
  - not always possible to intervene effectively;
  - nocturnal ventilation;
  - management of cachexia.

Fluid in the respiratory tree
- Causes:
  - secretions;
  - infection.
- Interventions:
  - antibiotics;
  - anticholinergics;

Effects of antibiotics and anticholinergics are mutually counterproductive. Anticholinergics reduce the volume of secretions but increase their viscosity, which may interfere with mucociliary clearance. Antibiotics may improve infection but carry their own adverse effects. The best approach needs individual assessment, taking into account priorities of the child and family.

Symptomatic pulmonary congestion due to cardiac failure may improve with diuretics.

Narrow airway
- Cause: pressure from tumour, reactive bronchoconstriction.
- Interventions:
  - steroids;
  - radiotherapy;
  - palliative chemotherapy;
  - stent.
- An element of reversible bronchoconstriction is not uncommon, even in terminal dyspnoea, and may be improved by β_2 agonists.
- Parenchymal metastatic lung disease is rarely symptomatic and does not usually need intervention.
- Management should be in close collaboration with paediatric oncology and radiotherapy colleagues.
- Long-term steroid therapy should usually be avoided.
- Surgical insertion of stent is invasive and often not appropriate.

Pain
- Causes:
  - metastatic bone disease in the ribs;
  - inflammation (e.g. pleuritic reaction);
  - rubbing of the ribs on the pelvis in extreme kyphoscoliosis.

Interventions

Good analgesic management using opioids and appropriate adjuvants such as NSAIDs, bisphosphonates, radiotherapy, etc.

Pneumothorax or effusion

- Cause: usually malignant.
- Surgical interventions:
  - analgesia;
  - pleural drainage;
  - pleurodesis.
- Pleural drainage in children usually demands admission to hospital and specialist anaesthetic and surgical involvement.
- Malignant effusions usually reaccumulate within a few days or, at most, weeks.
- Pleurodesis is painful in a significant minority of cases.
- Pleurodesis is unsuccessful in a significant minority of cases.

Cough and haemoptysis

- Causes:
  - infection;
  - tumour;
- Interventions for cough:
  - inhaled local anaesthetic agents have been used in adults, but are poorly tolerated in children and risk aspiration through impairment of the gag reflex;
  - opioids;
  - radiotherapy (see ➔ Interventions for haemoptysis below).
- Interventions for haemoptysis:
  - haemoptysis frightening for the child and family; should usually treat;
  - reassurance that a major haemorrhage is, in reality, unlikely;
  - radiotherapy has a dual effect of shrinking the tumour and reducing bleeding from the surface;
  - haemoptysis usually caused by a tumour pressing on a major airway; a parenchymal tumour or metastasis is rarely the cause;
  - etamsylate and tranexamic acid can both reduce the risk of haemoptysis;
  - prepare for the possibility of larger haemorrhage, including parenteral midazolam; ensure dark green surgical towels are by the child's bedside.

Upper airway secretions ('death rattle')

- Occurs in the last 24–48h of life.
- Usually occurs in a comatose patient who is unaware.
- Symptom is distressing for friends and family at the child's bedside and therefore should be treated.
- Interventions:
  - reduce any parenteral fluids to 50% maintenance; reassure the family that this will not in any way shorten the child's life;
  - anticholinergics (e.g. hyoscine patch or via sc syringe driver) reduce the volume, but increase the viscosity, of secretions;
  - suction can be uncomfortable in a child who is still aware but can be valued by the family as an intervention they can carry out.

Other causes of dyspnoea

Claustrophobia
- Causes:
  - inability to take a deep breath (e.g. due to muscle weakness);
  - presence of an oxygen mask on the face;
  - use of bi-level positive airways pressure (BiPAP) or non-invasive positive-pressure ventilation (NIPPV).
- Interventions:
  - movement of air on the face (e.g. open the window, switch on an electric fan);
  - consider the need for, or appropriateness of, a face mask.

Hypoxia
- Many and various causes, particularly in the final hours of life.
- Hypoxia should only be treated if symptomatic. Oxygen saturation monitors in the final days and weeks of life offer little benefit for most families.
- Oxygen does not relieve dyspnoea in the absence of hypoxaemia.[1]
- The need for oxygen in the palliative phase should be considered very carefully for the individual child and family.

Fear
The fear associated with difficulty in breathing leads to a powerful vicious cycle, in which difficulty in breathing reinforces anxiety, which, in turn, exacerbates difficulty in breathing. An ascending spiral of anxiety may result in a 'panic attack'.

Management

In developing a management strategy for dyspnoea, it is important to consider:

- subjective symptoms, as well as objective signs;
- non-pharmacological, as well as pharmacological, approaches;
- psychological, as well as physical, interventions.

Steps in managing dyspnoea

1. High index of suspicion. Consider the possibility of dyspnoea, and proactively ask about it.
2. Where practical, establish, in discussion with the child, whether breathing problems are a concern to himself or herself.
3. Explore what the breathing difficulties 'mean' to the child and family.
4. Take a careful history of the nature of the symptom.
5. Perform a careful examination.
6. Make a rational diagnosis of the cause(s) for dyspnoea.
7. Construct a rational therapeutic approach, weighing each intervention carefully, with respect to the potential good it may do and the potential harm.
8. Review the effectiveness of the intervention.

Interventions that do not depend on knowing the cause

- Adequate exploration of fears and, where appropriate, reassurance.
- Elementary breathing techniques aimed at putting the child and family back in control of the breathing.
- Breeze on the face, e.g. by opening the window, using an electric fan, or (if necessary) through a face mask.
- Complementary therapies (e.g. hypnosis).
- Opioids.[2] There are opioid receptors in the respiratory and cough centres of the brain. Doses of opioid effective for dyspnoea are ~50% of those required for pain. Otherwise, the principles of prescription and titration are precisely the same.
- Benzodiazepines. Benzodiazepines act on receptors in higher centres to relieve anxiety, and on receptors in the respiratory centre. Long-acting benzodiazepines, such as lorazepam and diazepam, can be useful for background dyspnoea. Buccal or parenteral midazolam is particularly useful for intervening in acute episodes of dyspnoea or panic attacks.
- Nebulized saline. Some patients derive benefit from nebulized saline. The mechanism is not clear but may be a combination of dilution of viscid secretions and the effect of blowing on the face.
- Other nebulized medications. The evidence for benefit of nebulized opioids in adults or in children is slight.[3] However, they do little or no harm, and individual patients sometimes report benefit. It is unclear whether this benefit is separable from that of blowing on the face. Nebulized mucolytics provide symptom benefit in cystic fibrosis.

Decision-making

- Because dyspnoea is a subjective symptom that correlates only poorly with observed abnormal parameters, it is critical to engage the child and family in a discussion, before embarking on a therapeutic strategy. All interventions carry the risk of adverse, as well as beneficial, effects, and it is not justifiable to commence an intervention to solve a problem that exists only in the eye of the observer.
- A special example of this is the use of NIPPV. There is now good evidence that this can improve symptoms and quality of life in many life-limited children.[4,5] Nevertheless, for some individual children and young people, the NIPPV itself is an intolerable burden.
- Like all palliative manoeuvres, NIPPV and other interventions for dyspnoea should be carried out only when the benefit to the patient (and sometimes the family) outweighs the burden.

References

1. Uronis, H.E., Currow, D.C., McCrory, D.C., Samsa, G.P., and Abernethy, A.P. (2008). Oxygen for relief of dyspnoea in mildly- or non-hypoxaemic patients with cancer: a systematic review and meta-analysis. *Br. J. Cancer* **98** (2), 294–9.
2. Hauer, J.M. (2015). Treating dyspnea with morphine sulfate in nonverbal children with neurological impairment. *Pediatr. Pulmonol.* **50** (4), E9–12.
3. Currow, D.C. and Abernethy, A.P. (2007). Pharmacological management of dyspnoea. *Curr. Opin. Support. Palliative Care* **1** (2), 96–101.
4. Mellies, U., Dohna-Schwake, C., Stehling, F., and Voit, T. (2004). Sleep disordered breathing in spinal muscular atrophy. *Neuromuscul. Disord.* **14** (12), 797–803.
5. Young, A.C., Wilson, J.W., Kotsimbos, T.C., and Naughton, M.T. (2008). Randomised placebo controlled trial of non-invasive ventilation for hypercapnia in cystic fibrosis. *Thorax* **63** (1), 72–7.

Chapter 12

Neurological symptoms

Epilepsy

Definition

Recurrent convulsive or non-convulsive seizures, caused by partial or generalized epileptogenic discharges in the cerebrum.

General points

- Not all seizures are grand-mal epileptic seizures; they come in many forms, and it is important to recognize the different types.
- Not all seizures require immediate administration of medication. The majority of seizures will settle, given 5–10min, particularly in children with neurodegenerative disorders.
- Look for the reversible causes of increased seizures, and attempt to correct them.
- Seizures can be very frightening for the child, family, and carers. Try to remain calm; give parents an explanation of what is happening, and treat the child in a logical manner.

Reversible causes of increased seizure frequency

- Infection.
- Renal failure.
- Hepatic failure.
- Electrolyte imbalance (sodium, calcium, or magnesium).
- Hypoglycaemia.
- Raised intracranial pressure.
- Inappropriate epilepsy management.
- Too rapid an increase or decrease of epilepsy medication.

General principles of management

- Correctly diagnose the type of epileptic seizure.[1–3]
- Know which drugs are used to treat the different types of seizures (Table 12.1).[4]
- Start with one drug, working up the dose gradually, until seizure control or side effects occur.[2]
- Add a second drug only if seizure control not achieved with the first drug alone.
- Remember to weigh up the benefits versus side effects of the treatments; 30% of children have behavioural problems, while on anticonvulsants.[5,6]
- Change doses gradually.
- Regular recalculation of drug dosage, as the child grows and puts on weight.
- Metabolism of drugs can be affected by hepatic and renal failure.[7]
- Children under the age of 3 years may need higher doses of drugs, due to their more efficient drug metabolism.
- Blood levels are generally unhelpful.
- If in doubt, ask a paediatric neurologist.

Table 12.1 Antiepileptic drugs*

Drugs	Advantages	Disadvantages	Comments
Carbamazepine	Effective for partial and tonic–clonic seizures, minimal side effects	Transient adverse effects during initiation; no parenteral formulation; may worsen absence seizures; complex pharmacokinetics. Drowsiness, coordination problems, and extrapyramidal movements	Drug of first choice for partial epilepsies
Ethosuximide	Effective for absence seizures; few side effects	Only for absence seizures; frequent gastrointestinal symptoms	First-choice drug for absence seizures
Phenobarbital	Broad spectrum of efficacy	Sedative, cognitive, or behavioural effects; hyperkinetic behaviour	Not first-choice drug, but safe and cheap; useful in cerebral irritation
Phenytoin	Effective: partial and tonic–clonic seizures; parenteral formulation	Cosmetic or dysmorphic side effects; saturation kinetics	Another first-choice drug for partial epilepsies; potent enzyme inhibitor
Primidone	Effective: partial and tonic–clonic seizures	Toxicity; behavioural effects, drowsiness, ataxia, personality changes	Not first-choice drug
Valproate (valproic acid)	Broad spectrum of efficacy	Weight gain, tremor, ataxia, drowsiness	First-choice drug for idiopathic epilepsy; an alternative for partial seizures
Gabapentin	Effective in partial and tonic–clonic seizures, well tolerated	Limited absorption, short half-life, moderate efficacy; somnolence	Mechanism of action unknown; additional use as adjuvant in neuropathic pain
Lamotrigine	Broad spectrum, sense of well-being	Hypersensitivity reaction rash, metabolism inducible; dizziness, ataxia, somnolence	
Vigabatrin	Effective: partial and tonic–clonic seizures, infantile spasms	Eye problems, dyskinesias	Unique mechanism of action

* Data from Mattson, R.H. (1996). The role of the old and the new antiepileptic drugs in special populations: mental and multiple handicaps. *Epilepsia* **37** (Suppl. 6), S45–53.

Intractable epilepsy

The management of intractable epilepsy is beyond the scope of this manual. However, it is worth remembering a few points.[2,8–12]

- 40% of children with intractable epilepsy are misdiagnosed. This can be due to:
  - an underlying aetiology overlooked;
  - misdiagnosis of the syndrome or seizure type;
  - poor EEG recording or interpretation;
  - non-epileptic disorders that mimic epileptic disorders.
- There are often errors in therapy due to:
  - inappropriate choice of drugs;
  - inappropriate dose and dosing interval;
  - inappropriate polytherapy.
- In all cases of intractable epilepsy, check:
  - that the child has actually seen a paediatric neurologist and has had a formal diagnosis of the type of epilepsy;
  - if on polytherapy, has this decision been made by a paediatric neurologist, and, if not, what is the rationale for the polytherapy?

Status epilepticus

Definition
When seizures occur so frequently that, over the course of 30 or more minutes, patients have not recovered from the coma produced by one attack, before the next attack supervenes.

Management
In the community or smaller units (major hospitals have established protocols that should be followed):[13]
- secure the airway;
- give oxygen;
- establish the cause;
- check for hypoglycaemia;
- If facilities available, check full blood count (FBC), urea and electrolytes (U & E), glucose, calcium, magnesium, liver function tests, and blood cultures. If possible, check the urine for infection.

First-line treatment
Diazepam
- iv: getting new access site is difficult, onset of action in 1–3min, effective in 80% of cases within 5min, short duration of action of 15–20min.
- Per rectum (pr): as a solution (suppositories take too long to work) works within 6–8min.
- NG tube or gastrostomy: best mode, if available.[14,15]

Midazolam
- Buccally: increasingly popular due to ease of administration, works within 6–8min.
- pr.[14–16]

Lorazepam
- iv: as infusion; give slowly to avoid apnoea.
- pr.
- Orally (po).
- Sublingually.

The metabolites of diazepam are active. Furthermore, diazepam accumulates in lipid stores. When these stores saturate, then the levels rise rapidly, leading to unexpected side effects (secondary peak phenomenon). This is not true of lorazepam.

Second-line treatment
If still fitting, then repeat the first-line treatment after 10–15min.

Third-line treatment
If there is still no response, then pr paraldehyde should be administered.

Paraldehyde should be mixed in an equal volume of arachis oil (or olive oil if there is any nut allergy), drawn up into a glass syringe, and given via a quill (if urgent, a plastic syringe can be used, provided it is drawn up and given immediately).

Fourth-line treatment
Hospitalize the child for advanced management, paralysis, and ventilation.

Terminal seizures or if not appropriate to hospitalize

In the terminal phase, seizures can become more severe and frequent. The child at this stage is normally not able to take or absorb oral anti-epileptics, and, in such cases, continuous sc midazolam or phenobarbital can be used. The physician needs to balance the heavily sedating effects of treatment against the benefits of seizure control. It may not be possible to control all the seizures, and it is necessary to explain to the parents that some minor seizures may break through and do not necessarily require escalation of treatment.

Midazolam subcutaneous infusion

- Onset of action 1–5min.
- Duration of action 1–5h.
- Easier to titrate than phenobarbital.
- Good anxiolytic.
- Dose can be steadily increased (up to 150mg/24h, then consider changing to phenobarbital).
- Only available in one strength, so volume in smaller Graseby syringe drivers can be a problem.
- Anecdotal evidence suggests that a small dose of diamorphine added to the syringe driver can help with seizures requiring increasing doses of midazolam.
- Clonazepam is an alternate to midazolam.[14–16]

Phenobarbital subcutaneous infusion

- Sedating.
- Anxiolytic.
- Do not combine with other drugs in syringe driver (only miscible with diamorphine and hyoscine).
- Should be diluted with water.

Spasticity

Definition
A condition of increased tone, spasms, clonus, weakness, and loss of dexterity.

Causes
- Cerebral palsy.
- Brain haemorrhage.
- Brain tumours.
- Anoxia.
- Vegetative state.

Management
- Multidisciplinary.[17]
- Physiotherapy.
- Surgical.
- Botulinum A injections.[18]
- Drugs:[19] not always very successful:
  - baclofen, po or by pump;
  - diazepam;
  - tizanidine;
  - dantrolene;
  - quinine;
  - gabapentin.

Myoclonus

Definition
Brief, abrupt, involuntary, non-suppressible, and jerky contractions, involving a single muscle or muscle group.[20]

Causes
- Normal; onset of sleep, exercise, anxiety.
- Neurodegenerative disorders.
- Secondary to opioid overdose.

Management
- Opioid rotation (see ➲ Chapter 6).
- Benzodiazepines:
  - diazepam;
  - lorazepam;
  - clonazepam.

Chorea

Definition
Frequent, brief, purposeless movements that tend to flow from body part to body part chaotically and unpredictably.[20]

Causes
- Rheumatic fever.
- Neurodegenerative disorder.
- Encephalopathy.
- Hypo- and hypernatraemia.
- Drugs, including:
  - haloperidol;
  - phenytoin;
  - phenothiazines.

Management
- Bed rest in a quiet, darkened room.
- Sodium valproate.

Dystonia

Definition
Syndrome of sustained muscle contractions, frequently causing twisting and repetitive movements or abnormal postures.[20]

Causes
- Neurodegenerative disorders.
- Metabolic disorders.
- In drug-induced reactions producing extrapyramidal reactions.
- Drugs, including:
  - dopamine antagonists;
  - antipsychotics;
  - antiemetics;
  - antidepressants;
  - anti-epileptics.

Management
- Anticholinergic drugs such as benztropine or diphenhydramine (in collaboration with the neurologist).
- Review medications, and reduce or stop drugs, if possible.

Akathisia

Definition

Motor restlessness, in which the patient feels compelled to pace up and down, or to change body position frequently.[20]

Causes

Drugs, including haloperidol and prochlorperazine.

Management

- Review medication, and reduce or stop drugs, if possible.
- Propranolol.

References

1. Shinnar, S. and Pellock, J.M. (2002). Update on the epidemiology and prognosis of pediatric epilepsy. *J. Child Neurol.* **17** (Suppl. 1), S4–17.
2. Udani, V. (2000). Evaluation and management of intractable epilepsy. *Indian J. Pediatr.* **67** (1 Suppl.), S61–70.
3. Murphy, J.V. and Dehkharghani, F. (1994). Diagnosis of childhood seizure disorders. *Epilepsia* **35** (Suppl. 2:), S7–17.
4. Mattson, R.H. (1996). The role of the old and the new antiepileptic drugs in special populations: mental and multiple handicaps. *Epilepsia* **37** (Suppl. 6), S45–53.
5. Dunn, D.W. (2003). Neuropsychiatric aspects of epilepsy in children. *Epilepsy Behav.* **4** (2), 101–6.
6. Holmes, G.L., Chevassus-Au-Lois, N., Sarkisian, M.R., and Ben-Ari, Y. (1997). [Consequences of recurrent seizures during development]. *Rev. Neurol.* **25** (141), 749–53.
7. Anderson, G.D. (2002). Children versus adults: pharmacokinetic and adverse-effect differences. *Epilepsia* **43** (Suppl. 3), 53–9.
8. Blume, W.T. (1992). Uncontrolled epilepsy in children. *Epilepsy Res. Suppl.* **5**, 19–24.
9. Camfield, P.R. and Camfield, C.S. (1996). Antiepileptic drug therapy: when is epilepsy truly intractable? *Epilepsia* **37** (Suppl. 1), S60–5.
10. Holmes, G.L. (1993). Seizure disorders in children. *Curr. Opin. Pediatr.* **5** (6), 653–9.
11. Iinuma, K. (1999). [General principles of treatment and effects of childhood intractable epilepsy]. *Rinsho Shinkeigaku* **39** (1), 75–6.
12. Steinborn, B. (2000). [Intractable epilepsy of childhood and its treatment]. *Neurol. Neurochir. Pol.* **33** (Suppl. 1), S60–5.
13. Mitchell, W.G. (1996). Status epilepticus and acute repetitive seizures in children, adolescents, and young adults: etiology, outcome, and treatment. *Epilepsia* **37** (Suppl. 1), S74–80.
14. Camfield, P.R. (1999). Buccal midazolam and rectal diazepam for treatment of prolonged seizures in childhood and adolescence: a randomised trial. *J. Pediatr.* **135** (3), 398–9.
15. Scott, R.C., Besag, F.M., and Neville, B.G. (1999). Buccal midazolam and rectal diazepam for treatment of prolonged seizures in childhood and adolescence: a randomised trial. *Lancet* **353** (9153), 623–6.
16. Grimshaw, D., Holyroyd, E., Anthony, D., and Hall, D.M. (1995). Subcutaneous midazolam, diamorphine and hyoscine infusion in palliative care of a child with neurodegenerative disease. *Child Care Health Dev.* **21** (6), 377–81.
17. Gormley, M.E., Jr., Krach, L.E., and Piccini, L. (2001). Spasticity management in the child with spastic quadriplegia. *Eur. J. Neurol.* **8** (Suppl. 5), 127–35.
18. Koman, L.A., Paterson Smith, B., and Balkrishnan, R. (2003). Spasticity associated with cerebral palsy in children: guidelines for the use of botulinum A toxin. *Paediatr. Drugs* **5** (1), 11–23.
19. Krach, L.E. (2001). Pharmacotherapy of spasticity: oral medications and intrathecal baclofen. *J. Child Neurol.* **16** (1), 31–6.
20. Schlaggar, B.L. and Mink, J.W. (2003). Movement disorders in children. *Pediatr. Rev.* **24** (2), 39–51.

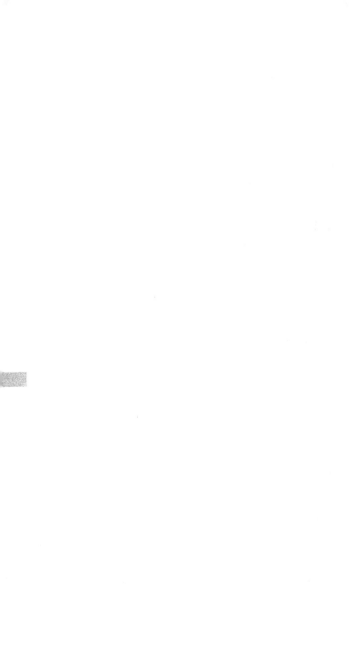

Psychological symptoms

Introduction

Disorders of the psyche (particularly depression and anxiety) are relatively common amongst children with life-limiting conditions. Most of the tools available for evaluating or assessing them in palliative medicine were developed for adults, as were strategies for treating them.[1]

Ideal practice is to collaborate with local child and adolescent mental health services in the management of all such children.[2] In many areas in the UK, service provision is such that this is rarely practical in children's palliative care. Nevertheless, where there is ready access to such services, advice should be sought.

Depression: general points

- Best clinical practice in managing depression in children was set out in 2005 by the National Institute for Health and Care Excellence (NICE).[2]
- Most evidence in relation to managing psychological symptoms is in the literature on child psychiatry and psychology, rather than in the context of paediatric palliative care.
- The standard *Diagnostic and Statistical Manual*, fourth edition (DSM-IV) and International classification of disease (ICD)-10 scales for assessing depression are inappropriate for assessing it in paediatric palliative care, because the clinical picture is dependent on the condition and developmental age of the child.
- Tools for diagnosing depression often do not take into account illness in the child.
- Clinicians may be reluctant to diagnose psychological problems,[3] as a result of:
  - concern over adding an additional burden of another condition on to the child and family;
  - belief that that reaction is normal under the circumstances of their existing condition;
  - lack of confidence in their own ability to diagnose and manage psychological problems;
  - belief that only an expert psychiatrist, psychologist, or counsellor can recognize this type of problem.
- Children with a life-limiting condition appear to report less depression than expected.
- Repression is a long-term behaviour pattern often manifest as a continually changing pattern of acceptance and denial. It can be a coping mechanism when dealing with their illness, particularly by adolescents.
- Children can have adjustment reactions (regression, enuresis, etc.) to serious illness, and it can be difficult to differentiate this from depression.
- The risk of developing psychological problems is linked to pre-existing psychosocial factors and maternal psychiatric/psychological state.

Managing depression

General principles
- Those working in paediatric palliative care should be familiar with the signs and symptoms of depression in children. The best tools for diagnosis are:
  - low threshold of suspicion;
  - listening to the child, family, and multidisciplinary team with care and compassion;
  - time, both in terms of the assessment, but also being prepared to talk when the child feels ready to open up; good care will require regular meetings with the child and family;
  - appropriately structured clinical interview.
- Be prepared to seek advice from a child psychiatrist, but it is not necessary for a doctor or specialist counsellor to tackle all the issues. The child may not choose to open up to the doctor but may well disclose their feelings to nurses, teachers, or religious leaders. It is important to support all these groups.
- Understand the stresses and strains in the family.
- Appreciate that the child may feel frightened and guilty about their illness and how it affects their family.
- Give honest answers to straight questions.
- Open communication and allowing the child to be involved in their management is very helpful.
- Medication only forms one part of the support that the child and family may need.
- Treatment should involve psychological therapies, including counselling and complementary therapies.
- Cognitive behavioural therapy has been shown to be very effective in the normal paediatric population, but its benefit in life-limited children is mainly anecdotal.
- Depression and anxiety are often interlinked, so assessment must encompass both.

Pharmacological approach
- Tricyclic antidepressants and selective serotonin re-uptake inhibitors (SSRIs).
- The safety and efficacy of drugs used in the treatment of depression in children has not been established; long-term safety information is also lacking.[4]
- The use of antidepressants is determined by the individual child's medical condition, medications, psychiatric state, and risk of suicide.
- Initiation of treatment should be made after open and honest discussion with the child, family, and care team. Very few children or parents will say no to medication, if it is truly required.
- Rapid withdrawal of any antidepressant can cause nausea, vomiting, anorexia, headaches, and giddiness. Any child on medication for over 8 weeks should have this withdrawn slowly.

Tricyclic antidepressants
- Dosages for antidepressant benefit have to be sufficiently high; however, at that level, side effects often limit their benefit.
- These can be split into two groups: sedating (amitriptyline) and non-sedating (imipramine).
- The main concerns centre around antimuscarinic and cardiac side effects.
- Side effects include:
  - arrhythmias;
  - heart block;
  - convulsions—use with caution in epilepsy;
  - drowsiness;
  - dry mouth;
  - blurred vision;
  - constipation;
  - urinary retention;
  - suicidal thoughts/behaviour.

Selective serotonin re-uptake inhibitors
- The Committee on Safety of Medicines (CSM) has advised that the risk and benefit balance for the following SSRIs is considered unfavourable in the under 18 year olds: citalopram, escitalopram, paroxetine, and sertraline.[5,6]
- Only fluoxetine has shown to be effective in treating depression in children.[7]
- The risk from SSRIs appears to be related to suicidal thoughts and behaviour (there have been no confirmed deaths). This risk is particularly high in the first few weeks of treatment.
- Hyponatraemia has been associated with antidepressants (particularly SSRIs). This should be considered in any child who develops unexpected drowsiness, confusion, or convulsions, while on antidepressants.
- SSRIs can cause an increase in anxiety in the first 2–4 weeks of treatment.
- It can take up to 4 weeks to see an improvement in a child, and up to 6–8 weeks to see maximum benefit from the medication.
- Use with caution in children with epilepsy, cardiac disease, diabetes mellitus, history of mania, or bleeding disorders.
- Side effects are similar to those of tricyclics, but there tend to be less sedating and fewer antimuscarinic effects, although nausea and anxiety are greater in the first few weeks.

Anxiety

General points
- Anxiety can come from a number of different sources:[8]
  - separation anxiety;
  - procedure-related;
  - death anxiety;
  - inpatient admission (abandonment);
  - receiving bad news.
- As with depression, doctors may be reluctant to diagnose, as they see the behaviour as normal under the circumstances.
- Diagnostic tools tend to be unhelpful.
- Maternal psychiatric disorder increases the risk of anxiety in the child.
- Over the development age of 10 years, almost all children are aware of their prognosis, whether they have been told by parents/doctors or not.[9]
- Anxiety is significantly reduced if the child is openly told, in terms they understand, about their condition.
- Death anxiety is greatest in children whose development age is between 6 and 10 years.

General principles of management
(See ➲ Chapter 13, Managing depression, pp. 126–7.)
- Good communication skills and allowing the child to express their anxiety are important.
- Music therapy, art therapy, massage, reflexology, hypnosis, and acupuncture have all been shown to be very effective in managing a range of different types of anxiety.
- Cognitive behavioural therapy has been shown to be effective in the normal paediatric population, but its benefits in paediatric palliative care have only been shown in procedural pain.
- Look at the developmental age of the child when assessing symptoms.
- Remember to treat the family, as well as the child.

Pharmacological approach
- Benzodiazepines are the main group of drugs used to treat short-term anxiety.[10]
- The type of benzodiazepine used is dependent on the nature and type of anxiety symptoms.
- They are best used as short-term treatments.
- For more chronic anxiety states, antidepressant medication should be used.
- Benzodiazepines are particularly helpful in the first few weeks when SSRIs are started.

Benzodiazepines
Midazolam
- Fast- and short-acting (<1h).
- Can be given by the sc, po, or buccal route. Intranasal route was once popular but can cause nasal irritation and has been superseded in most places by buccal.
- Is particularly useful in the acutely anxious dying child or for procedural anxiety.
- Can be given as a continuous infusion.
- Rarely causes paradoxical agitation.

Lorazepam
- Long-acting (around 8–12h).
- Can be given by the sublingual, po, or pr route.
- The injection solution can be used for the sublingual or pr route.
- The tablet is particularly useful in the older child, as it is easy to carry around and can be used po or sublingually.
- Is particularly useful in the acutely anxious dying child or for procedural anxiety.

Diazepam
- Slow-acting when taken orally.
- Longer-acting than midazolam or lorazepam.
- Can develop cumulative effect where repeated dosages can cause sudden heavy sedation.

Other drugs for anxiety
- Fluoxetine has been used for generalized anxiety.[11]
- Pregabalin has been used effectively in adults with generalized anxiety, but there is no evidence in paediatric palliative care.[12]

Insomnia

Insomnia is a problem not only for the child, but also the parents.

Causes

It is important to address the possible causes for insomnia, before embarking on medication:

- fear and/or anxiety;
- underlying depression;
- disturbed night-time routine from giving medication or conducting procedures;
- pain, discomfort, or side effects of medication or feeding;
- altered biorhythms with the child sleeping during the day due to medication causing sedation or child's/family's routine (e.g. parents putting the child to sleep during the day, so they can have a break);
- the disease process itself; many neurodegenerative conditions are linked to altered or diminished sleep patterns.

General principles of management

- Identify anxiety or depression, and manage appropriately.
- Look at the sleep pattern, and try to devise a routine before bedtime to help relax the child down such as warm bath, story, darkened room, etc.
- Alter drug timing to reduce night disturbances as much as possible.
- Change any medication that may cause problems in the night (e.g. NSAIDs and dyspepsia at night).
- Consider complementary therapies, such as aromatherapy or massage, for both the child and also the parents.
- Develop a realistic expectation of how long the child can, or needs to, sleep with the parents.
- Accept that adolescents may choose to go to sleep very late at night and sleep in.

Pharmacological approach

The use of medication should be considered as a last resort for insomnia when all other approaches have failed. A number of different drugs can be used for insomnia.

Chloral

- Chloral hydrate was formerly a popular hypnotic in children.
- Large volumes and gastric irritation limit its usefulness.
- Chloral derivatives are soporific (i.e. promote sleep), but not anxiolytic.[13]

Temazepam

- A long-acting benzodiazepine now used extensively, particularly for the older child.
- Works for 4–6h.
- Should be taken up to 1h before bedtime.

Promethazine
- An antihistamine.
- Sedative effects can diminish after a few days of continued use.

Melatonin
- A pineal hormone that affects sleep patterns.
- Used for sleep disorder in children with cerebral palsy, attention-deficit disorder, and autism.
- Increasingly being tried out of licence for children with neurodegenerative conditions.
- Should be initiated and supervised by specialists.[14,15]

Terminal delirium

Delirium, often called acute confusion state, can be seen at any stage through a child's illness but is more prevalent at the terminal stage.

Clinical features
- Terminal restlessness.
- Acute onset.
- Fluctuating nature.
- Disorientation.
- Agitation or lethargy.
- Altered perception.
- Auditory or visual hallucinations.
- Potentially reversible.

Causes
- Drugs:
  - opioids;
  - antimuscarinics;
  - corticosteroids.
- Drug withdrawal.
- Cerebral disease:
  - hypoxia;
  - sepsis;
  - primary or secondary cancers;
  - cerebral vascular accident.
- Anxiety or depression.
- Pain.
- Constipation.
- Organ failure:
  - liver;
  - kidney.
- Biochemical:
  - hypercalcaemia;
  - hyponatraemia;
  - hyperosmolality.
- Infection:
  - urinary;
  - respiratory;
  - neurological;
  - other causes of septicaemia.
- Nutritional deficiencies.

General principles of management
- Assess fully; identify reversible causes, and manage appropriately.
- Reassure the family and the child by explaining what is happening.
- Repeat important information to the child.
- Set a calm environment for the child:
  - reduce noise;
  - adequate lighting;

- have the family around the child;
- use familiar staff to care for the child;
- use bedding, toys, and comfort items with which the child is familiar.
- Do not use any forms of restraint.

Pharmacological approach

From the onset, it is important to establish what you hope to achieve with medication. The plan should be to help improve the mental state, while controlling sedation. This is not always achievable.

- There is no research available for the use of drugs to manage delirium in paediatric palliative care. Treatments used are extrapolated from adult palliative care.
- Two main groups of drugs are used—phenothiazines and benzodiazepines—but phenobarbital also deserves a special mention.

Phenothiazines

- Haloperidol is the drug of choice in delirium.[16]
  - It is a potent neuroleptic with antidopaminergic activity.
  - It has relative few anticholinergic side effects.
  - Extrapyramidal reactions occur rarely at higher doses.
  - It improves cognition.
  - It has sedative effects at higher doses.
  - It can be given by the po, sc, iv, or im route.
  - It is fast-acting within hours.
  - It combines with benzodiazepines for rapid sedation.
- Levomepromazine.
  - It is a potent neuroleptic with antidopaminergic activity.
  - Used as an antiemetic in children.
  - In higher doses, it can be used to induce sedation.

Benzodiazepines

- Midazolam or lorazepam are the drugs of choice.
- They should not be used alone, as they may worsen delirium.[17]
- They do not improve cognition but only induce sedation.
- They combine well with haloperidol.
- They can be given by the po, sublingual, buccal, pr, sc, or iv route.
- At higher doses, they can cause paradoxical agitation and delirium.
- Children with neurodegenerative disorders are already often on benzodiazepines for their epilepsy, and these children can tolerate high doses of benzodiazepines.

Phenobarbital

- Phenobarbital can be used as second-line treatment.
- It can help control symptoms of agitation.
- Particularly good if anticonvulsant action required.
- Elevates seizure threshold (phenothiazines lower threshold).
- If used as sc infusion, it should be used as sole agent, with regular assessment of the insertion site, as it can cause skin irritation.[18]

References

1. Kelly, B., McClement, S., and Chochinov, H.M. (2006). Measurement of psychological distress in palliative care. *Palliat. Med.* **20** (8), 779–89.
2. National Institute for Health and Care Excellence (2005). *Depression in children and young people: identification and management.* NICE CG28. National Institute for Health and Care Excellence, London.
3. Froese, A.P. (1977). Pediatric referrals to psychiatry: III. Is the psychiatrist's opinion heard? *Int. J. Psychiatry Med.* **8** (3), 295–301.
4. Paediatric Formulary Committee (2015). *BNF for children (BNFC) 2015–2016.* Pharmaceutical Press, London.
5. Hetrick, S.E., Merry, S.N., McKenzie, J., Sindahl, P., and Proctor, M. (2007). Selective serotonin reuptake inhibitors (SSRIs) for depressive disorders in children and adolescents. *Cochrane Database Syst. Rev.* **3**, CD004851.
6. Whittington, C.J., Kendall, T., Fonagy, P., Cottrell, D., Cotgrove, A., and Boddington, E. (2004). Selective serotonin reuptake inhibitors in childhood depression: systematic review of published versus unpublished data. *Lancet* **363** (9418), 1341–5.
7. Emslie, G.J., Kennard, B.D., Mayes, T.L., Nightingale-Teresi, J., Carmody, T., Hughes, C.W., et al. (2008). Fluoxetine versus placebo in preventing relapse of major depression in children and adolescents. *Am. J. Psychiatry* **165** (4), 459–67.
8. Hart, D. and Bossert, E. (1994). Self-reported fears of hospitalized school-age children. *J. Pediatr. Nurs.* **9** (2), 83–90.
9. Spinetta, J.J., Rigler, D., and Karon, M. (1973). Anxiety in the dying child. *Pediatrics* **52** (6), 841–5.
10. Ashton, H. (1994). Guidelines for the rational use of benzodiazepines. When and what to use. *Drugs* **48** (1), 25–40.
11. Birmaher, B., Axelson, D.A., Monk, K., Kalas, C., Clark, D.B., Ehmann, M., et al. (2003). Fluoxetine for the treatment of childhood anxiety disorders. *J. Am. Acad. Child Adolesc. Psychiatry* **42** (4), 415–23.
12. Alvarez, E., Olivares, J.M., Carrasco, J.L., Lopez-Gomez, V., and Rejas, J. (2015). Clinical and economic outcomes of adjunctive therapy with pregabalin or usual care in generalized anxiety disorder patients with partial response to selective serotonin reuptake inhibitors. *Ann. Gen. Psychiatry* **14** (1), 2.
13. Jones, D.P. and Jones, E.A. (1963). Drugs for insomnia. *Can. Med. Assoc. J.* **89**, 1331.
14. Smits, M.G., van Stel, H.K., van der Heijden, K., Meijer, A.M., Coenen, A.M., and Kerkhof, G.A. (2003). Melatonin improves health status and sleep in children with idiopathic chronic sleep-onset insomnia: a randomized placebo-controlled trial. *J. Am. Acad. Child Adolesc. Psychiatry* **42** (11), 1286–93.
15. Zhdanova, I.V. (2005). Melatonin as a hypnotic: pro. *Sleep Med. Rev.* **9** (1), 51–65.
16. Breitbart, W. and Strout, D. (2000). Delirium in the terminally ill. *Clin. Geriatr. Med.* **16** (2), 357–72.
17. Breitbart, W., Marotta, R., Platt, M.M., Weisman, H., Deverenco, M., Grau, C., et al. (1996). A double-blind trial of haloperidol, chlorpromazine, and lorazepam in the treatment of delirium in hospitalized AIDS patients. *Am. J. Psychiatry* **153** (2), 231–7.
18. Stirling, L.C., Kurowska, A., and Tookman, A. (1999). The use of phenobarbitone in the management of agitation and seizures at the end of life. *J. Pain Symptom Manage.* **17** (5), 363–8.

Skin symptoms

Epidermolysis bullosa

Definition

Epidermolysis bullosa (EB) is a rare (1 in 17 000 births) genetic condition that leads to fragile skin. It is characterized as a group of varying genetic disorders that produce blisters and shearing with minimal pressure or injury.

General points

- Dependent on the type, children can have blisters anywhere on their skin or in the gastrointestinal tract.
- The lung, heart, and renal tract can all be involved.
- Many children have anaemia and malnutrition problems.
- There are three distinct types of EB.[1]

Epidermolysis bullosa simplex

- Most common type, affecting 65–70% of all children with EB.
- Histologically shows lack of adhesion of the skin above the basement membrane.
- Inherited as a dominant trait; often parents have a family history of the condition (rarely due to gene mutation).
- Blisters affect the hands and feet, although a rarer form can occur over the whole body.
- Most children will survive well into adulthood.
- Children can be born with severe blistering, but it invariably improves with time.
- Made worse by heat.

Junctional epidermolysis bullosa

- Most aggressive form, affecting 5–10% of all children with EB.
- Histologically shows lack of adhesion of the skin through the basement membrane.
- Inherited recessively. Unexpected diagnosis for parents.
- Most serious type is the Herlitz form.
- 50% die within the first 2 years of life. The other 50% of children have a milder form and can do well.
- Children can develop severe systemic problems.
  - Gastrointestinal: blistering throughout the gastrointestinal tract, making eating painful. Gastro-oesophageal reflux can lead to oesophageal strictures. Malnutrition with anaemia is common. NG tubes and gastrostomies can cause their own problems with the skin. Perianal blisters can cause pain on defecation and lead to constipation.
  - Anaemia: due to malnutrition and chronic blood loss from the skin and mucosa.
  - Respiratory: bullae formation in the larynx leads to a hoarse cry and stridor.
  - Cardiac: rarely, some children can develop fatal dilated cardiomyopathy.
  - Renal: occurs rarely.

Dystrophic epidermolysis bullosa

- This type of EB derives its name from the fact that the blistering associated with the condition tends to heal with scar formation.
- Affects 25% of all children with EB.
- Children histologically show lack of adhesion of the skin below the basement membrane.
- Can be inherited as a dominant or recessive trait.
- There is wide variation in the severity of dystrophic EB.
- The mildest type (the dominant form) can allow an almost normal life. Unfortunately, this group has a high risk of developing squamous cell carcinoma of the skin before the age of 35 years. The average life expectancy after tumour diagnosis is 5 years.
- Most serious type is the recessive form known as Hallopeau–Siemens.
- Children with the more aggressive form of dystrophic EB can develop severe systemic problems similar to those of junctional EB. In addition, children with dystrophic EB can also have problems with:
  - skin: scarring leads to severe contractures, most notably to the hands;
  - gastrointestinal: scarring in the mouth can lead to the tongue becoming fused to the base of the mouth and subsequently loss of the labial sulcus and microstomia; webs and strictures can form in the oesophagus;
  - renal: nephropathy and chronic post-infectious glomerulonephritis can occur.

Managing epidermolysis bullosa

The management of EB requires a multidisciplinary approach, organized and coordinated by specialized units. In the UK, this would be via Great Ormond Street Hospital or Birmingham Children's Hospital.

- The first and foremost part of the management is to make the correct diagnosis by skin biopsy assessed by a unit specializing in this type of histopathology.
- Then the issues of handling, dressings, and symptom management need to be addressed.

Handling

- Because skin will break down with minimal pressure or shearing force, handling should be kept to a minimum.
- Babies and small infants should be lifted, using the roll and lift technique (rolled to one side, and then one hand on the buttocks and the other on the head or neck).
- No children with EB should be lifted under their arms.
- Children should be cuddled gently as, due to hyperalgesia, they can experience pain from this.
- Children can be kissed gently.
- Older children may prefer to move themselves.
- Children with some types of EB can attend normal schools, but there needs to be pre-planning, in terms of teaching assistants, leaving classes early or late to avoid being bumped or knocked, etc.
- Bathing for some children may be impossible due to pain.

Dressings

- Dressing changing can be a painful experience. This is due to pain from the skin lesions, hyperalgesia, and sometimes anticipatory pain.
- Correct non-adherent dressings should be used.
- Dressing changing should be kept to a minimum.
- Adequate analgesia should be used.
- Dressing changing should be done as quickly as possible, as exposure of the wounds can be painful.

Pain

- The management of pain follows the same principles as discussed in Chapters 4 to 7, but there are particular issues associated with procedural pain.[2]
- Non-pharmacological modalities, such as physiotherapy and visualization, can be very helpful.
- For mild pain from minor dressing changes, paracetamol or NSAIDs can be used.
- For more severe pain, Entonox®, fentanyl lozenges, or morphine given in sufficient time can be used.
- Anxiety may require a small dose of benzodiazepines such as lorazepam or midazolam.
- Background pain can be managed with slow-release morphine.
- The neuropathic component of pain associated with EB responds well to amitriptyline or gabapentin.
- In the terminal phase, a syringe driver can be used.[3]

Pruritus

Definition

An unpleasant sensation that provokes a desire to scratch.

Pathophysiology

- Arises in the skin, conjunctivae, and mucous membranes.
- Can be classified as:[4]
  - cutaneous: arises from the skin;
  - neuropathic: damage to nerves or by direct irritation;
  - psychological.
- Transmitted through C fibres (similar to pain).
- Receptors are more superficial than pain receptors.
- Fibres respond to pruritogens, including histamine, acetylcholine, and peripheral serotonin.
- Pruritus increases with heat, anxiety, and boredom.

Causes

- Opioids particularly can cause pruritus, and this is more common in children than adults.
- Drugs: many drugs can cause problems, but particularly antibiotics (penicillin) and anti-epileptics (phenytoin).
- Eczema or dry skin.
- Scabies or lice.
- Renal failure.
- Hepatic disease causing jaundice.
- Haematological disorders, particularly leukaemias and lymphomas.
- Acquired immune deficiency syndrome (AIDS).
- Psychological.

Management

- Look at the possible causes, and treat appropriately.
- Simple rehydration of the skin with moisturizers.
- Cut back nails, with or without the use of mittens.
- Pruritus decreases with cold, distraction, and relaxation.
- Keep the child cool.
- The child should wear loose-fitting cotton clothes.
- Calamine lotion.
- If the skin is inflamed, then use mild steroid creams such as hydrocortisone.
- Oral corticosteroids can be used if the skin is very inflamed or for pruritus in terminal Hodgkin's lymphoma.
- NSAIDs can help by reducing prostaglandins, which can sensitize nerve endings to pruritogenic substances.
- H_1 antihistamines are used extensively in most types of pruritus, but understanding the pathophysiology of pruritus clearly indicates that there will be occasions when they are poorly effective or completely ineffective.
- Serotonin antagonist (e.g. ondansetron) can relieve some types of opioid-induced[5] and cholestatic pruritus.

Fungating tumours

General points
- Fungating tumours are rare in children.
- Fungating tumours occur when a primary or secondary tumour invades through the skin, leading to breakdown and ulceration of the skin.
- The tumour may spread locally or break down into a cavity.
- The resulting necrosis of the tissue may then become infected, bleed, or discharge an exudate.
- In children, the issues around disfigurement, body image, and smell may cause considerable psychological problems.

Causes
- Rhabdomyosarcoma.
- Nerve sheath tumours (e.g. complicating neurofibromatosis).
- Squamous cell carcinoma.
- Lymphoma.

Management
- Treat reversible factors:
  - improve nutrition;
  - stop or reduce steroids.
- Modify the appearance of the tumour:
  - surgery by debulking;
  - radiotherapy;
  - chemotherapy.
- Control pain:
  - during dressing changes, consider Entonox®, fentanyl lozenge, po or buccal morphine or diamorphine;
  - localized pain: consider topical diamorphine soaked into a dressing or topical anaesthetic agents such as lidocaine;
  - chronic pain: use slow-release morphine.
- Exudates:
  - use appropriate dressings (Table 14.1).
- Odour:
  - a counter-odour, e.g. household air freshener or aromatherapy oils;
  - a deodorant, e.g. ostomy deodorizers or electric deodorizer;
  - metronidazole, either topically or systemically, to treat anaerobic organisms;
  - live yoghurt;
  - charcoal-impregnated dressings;
  - occlusive dressings, either OpSite® (total) or Granuflex® (almost total);
  - honey and icing sugar dressings.
- If haemorrhage is a problem:
  - topical adrenaline 1 in 1000;
  - calcium alginate dressings have haemostatic properties;
  - radiotherapy;
  - use non-adherent dressings, and soak off with normal saline.
- If surrounding skin at risk from exudate:
  - protect with barrier ointment.

Pressure sores

General points

This is one symptom in which there is universal agreement with the adage 'prevention is better than cure'.

- Continual assessment of the skin is essential in all children with life-limiting conditions. This should not be just a nursing duty but should be part of the regular medical check of all children by doctors.
- Paediatric nurses often have very limited experience of managing pressure sores. It is often helpful to involve specialist wound care nurses from the adult world, as the principles of treatment are the same.
- It is important to make dressings cosmetically acceptable to the child.
- Try to remove dressings with minimal pain.
- Try to lengthen the time between dressing changes.
- Cost-effectiveness of the different types of dressings should be appreciated.
- The Braden Q Scale for assessing risk of pressure sores in the paediatric population is the best validated of all the scales, but even this scale is not completely accurate for children in the acute hospital setting.[6,7]

Risk factors

The risk factors associated with developing pressure sores are:[8]

- tissue ischaemia by external pressure sufficient to overcome capillary pressure;
- sensory perception;
- skin moisture;
- activity;
- mobility;
- risk of friction and shear;
- nutritional status;
- incontinence.

Staging

A staging system has been devised and is helpful in the management of pressure sores:[9]

- stage 1: intact skin, but erythema present;
- stage 2: partial skin damage to the epidermis and dermis;
- stage 3: full-thickness damage down to the subcutaneous tissue;
- stage 4: extensive damage down to underlying structures such as muscle or tendon.

Managing pressure sores

- Prevention with early aggressive intervention.
- Monitor pressure points.
- Regular turning.
- Pressure-relieving measures:
  - appropriate mattresses, air beds being the best;
  - pressure-relieving cushions.

- Assess and manage the child's nutritional status. Dietitians are particularly useful.
- Maintain good skin care with good hygiene and hydration.

Table 14.1 lists the types of dressings and their uses.[10]
- For stage 1 pressure sore:
  - use occlusive dressing/films to protect the sore;
  - be careful when removing not to cause further traumatic damage to the surrounding skin.
- For healing ulcers undergoing epithelialization:
  - film dressings;
  - low adherent dressings;
  - hydrocolloid interactive dressings.
- For light exudate:
  - film dressings;
  - hydrocolloid interactive dressings;
  - low adherent dressings;
  - alginate dressings;
  - hydrophilic foam dressings.
- For heavy exudate:
  - hydrocolloid interactive dressings;
  - hydrogel with secondary dressings;
  - alginate dressings;
  - hydrophilic foam dressings;
  - use of paediatric stoma bag.
- For cavities:
  - alginate cavity dressing;
  - silastic foam if the wound is clean;
  - foam dressing.
- If debridement is required:
  - surgery;
  - enzymes;
  - hydrocolloid paste with dressing;
  - hydrogel.

Table 14.1 Types of dressing and their uses

Type	Common names	Notes
Films	OpSite®, Tegaderm®	Allow observation; cannot absorb exudate
Low adherent	Release®, Mepore®	Absorbs some exudate
Hydrocolloids	Granuflex®, Comfeel®, DuoDerm®	May be left for up to 1 week
Hydrogels	IntraSite® Gel, Iodosorb®	Absorb large amounts of exudate
Alginates	Kaltostat®, Sorbsan®	Haemostatic
Foams	Lyofoam®, Silastic®	For cavities

- If the wound is infected:
  - topical metronidazole;
  - irrigate the wound with iv metronidazole solution;
  - systemic antibiotics;
  - honey and icing sugar dressings.

References

1. Fine, J.D., Eady, R.A., Bauer, E.A., Briggaman, R.A., Bruckner-Tuderman, L., Christiano, A., et al. (2000). Revised classification system for inherited epidermolysis bullosa: Report of the Second International Consensus Meeting on diagnosis and classification of epidermolysis bullosa. *J. Am. Acad. Dermatol.* **42** (6), 1051–66.
2. Herod, J., Denyer, J., Goldman, A., and Howard, R. (2002). Epidermolysis bullosa in children: pathophysiology, anaesthesia and pain management. *Paediatr. Anaesth.* **12** (5), 388–97.
3. O'Neill, B., Lucas, C., and Gannon, C. (2001). Use of a subcutaneous syringe driver in epidermolysis bullosa. *Palliat. Med.* **15** (1), 77–8.
4. Twycross, R., Greaves, M.W., Handwerker, H., Jones, E.A., Libretto, S.E., Szpietowski, J.C., et al. (2003). Itch: scratching more than the surface. *Q. J. Med.* **96** (1), 7–26.
5. Kyriakides, K., Hussain, S.K., and Hobbs, G.J. (1999). Management of opioid-induced pruritus: a role for 5-HT3 antagonists? *Br. J. Anaesth.* **82** (3), 439–41.
6. Quigley, S.M. and Curley, M.A. (1996). Skin integrity in the pediatric population: preventing and managing pressure ulcers. *J. Soc. Pediatr. Nurs.* **1** (1), 7–18.
7. Pallija, G., Mondozzi, M., and Webb, A.A. (1999). Skin care of the pediatric patient. *J. Pediatr. Nurs.* **14** (2), 80–7.
8. Bergstrom, N., Braden, B.J., Laguzza, A., and Holman, V. (1987). The Braden scale for predicting pressure sore risk. *Nurs. Res.* **36** (4), 205–10.
9. National Pressure Ulcer Advisory Panel (1992). *Statement on pressure ulcer prevention.* Agency for Health Care Policy and Research, Reston, Virginia. Available at: http://www.npuap.org/positn1.htm.
10. Twycross, R.G. and Wilcock, A. (2001). *Symptom management in advanced cancer*, third edition. Radcliffe Medical Press, Abingdon.

Chapter 15

Palliative care emergencies

Introduction

What is a 'palliative care emergency'?

A good working definition is a symptom situation that is serious and demands immediate and skilled specialist attention, but is also unusual enough for there to be a possibility that the specialist has not often encountered it.

In a palliative care emergency, the patient experiences sudden and severe distress that can only be relieved by prompt and confident intervention by the palliative care team. There is little time to prepare for it, and, to the specialist in PPM, an emergency is defined by the importance of already having a clear strategy for dealing with it. That can be challenging for those working in paediatric palliative care, because most are rare. They should make themselves thoroughly familiar with the theoretical management of emergencies, even if they have not yet had to manage them in practice.

The key principles to managing palliative care emergencies are the following.
- Anticipate that they may happen.
- Recognize early that they are happening.
- Have a plan ready for when they do happen.

PPM emergencies should always be managed by the tertiary PPM team, where one is available, or in collaboration with a specialist adult palliative medicine team otherwise.

There are six emergencies:
- cord compression;
- catastrophic haemorrhage;
- severe uncontrolled pain;
- superior vena cava (SVC) obstruction;
- intestinal obstruction;
- hypercalcaemia.

Cord compression

Pathophysiology
- Usually a complication of cancer.
- Can occur as a result of soft tissue expansion or sudden vertebral collapse.
- In children, acute cord compression rare.

Signs and symptoms
- Classically, sudden onset of back pain.
- Neurological symptoms, particularly loss of bladder or bowel control.
- Sudden and unexplained lack of mobility.
- In children, onset typically more insidious than in adults, and classic symptoms and signs may not appear.

Management
- Depends on the situation.
- Reduction of tumour oedema through high-dose dexamethasone.
- Reduction of tumour mass through radiation or emergency debulking surgery.
- Outcome for neurological recovery is poor if symptoms have been present for more than 48h.
- In practice, cord compression in children is typically non-acute, and it is rare for neurological recovery to be possible in the palliative situation.
- Invasive interventions, such as surgery, are usually not appropriate in children.

Catastrophic haemorrhage

Pathophysiology
- Usually complicates tumours close to, or eroding through, a major vessel.
- In reality, very rare.
- Greatly feared by families and patients.

Signs and symptoms
- May complicate lymphopoietic conditions, such as leukaemia, in which platelet numbers and function are both reduced.
- Often preceded by oozing, epistaxis, or haemoptysis.
- Correlation of platelet numbers with risk of haemorrhage is poor, and platelet numbers alone should not be an indication for transfusion.

Management
- Be aware of the possibility, and anticipate it.
- Platelet transfusions, tranexamic acid, and etamsylate to optimize clotting.
- Soften the impact by discussion with the family, and provision of green towels against which blood is less obvious should haemorrhage occur.
- Arrange for a parenteral quick-acting anxiolytic, such as midazolam, and analgesics, such as diamorphine, to be by the patient's bedside, in case haemorrhage should occur.

Severe uncontrolled pain

Pathophysiology
- Rare in PPM.
- Often results from inexpert opioid titration and adjuvant prescription in early stages of pain.
- Always has a major anxiety and fear component.

Signs and symptoms
- Pain suddenly becoming worse, often with no obvious cause.
- Apparent ineffectiveness even of large doses of opioids.

Management
- Involve the specialist palliative care team as soon as the diagnosis is made.
- Use the parenteral route to secure control as soon as possible.
- Palliative care team will administer a slow injection of opioid until pain goes.
- Calculation of regular and breakthrough opioid doses is made on basis of the dose required to control pain.

Superior vena cava obstruction

Pathophysiology
- Venous obstruction in the mediastinum and upper chest.
- Usual cause is tumour, particularly lymphoma.
- Pulmonary congestion leads to dyspnoea.
- Congestion of intracranial vessels leads to feeling of fullness and headache.

Signs and symptoms
- Headache, pressure, or 'fullness' in the head, worse on sneezing or bending forwards.
- Shortness of breath and discomfort in the chest.
- Facial plethora, obvious collateral vessels over the upper chest wall.

Management
- Management of individual symptoms (particularly pain and dyspnoea).
- Reduction of tumour oedema using steroids (use in discussion with oncologists, as some lymphomas may be very sensitive to steroids).
- Reduction of tumour mass using radiotherapy.
- Surgical insertion of stent into the SVC.

Intestinal obstruction

Pathophysiology
- Obstruction leads to proximal dilatation.
- Dilatation leads to stretching of the gut wall.
- Stretching of the gut wall leads to increased secretion.
- Increased secretion exacerbates dilatation.
- Relatively rare in children.
- May occur with abdominal tumours, such as neuroblastoma, or where there is abdominal extension of pelvic tumours.

Signs and symptoms
- Nausea and vomiting.
- Constipation.
- Severe intermittent colicky abdominal pain.
- Abdominal dilatation.
- Usually occurring in context of a known abdominal tumour.

Management
- Surgery sometimes an option if a single discrete obstruction.
- Reduce spasm (anticholinergics, e.g. hyoscine hydrobromide).
- Strong analgesia (e.g. diamorphine).
- Antiemetics (e.g. haloperidol).
- Reduce secretions (reduce fluid intake; nil by mouth; consider octreotide).
- Consider prokinetics (e.g. metoclopramide) if obstruction is not complete, such that there is the possibility of spontaneous resolution.
- Consider steroids to reduce tumour oedema.

Prokinetics and anticholinergics are mutually inhibitory and should not usually be used together. As many as half of all intestinal obstructions associated with malignant disease may resolve spontaneously, without the need for surgical intervention.

Hypercalcaemia

Pathophysiology
- Extremely rare in children, as associated with adult cancers such as breast, thyroid, and prostate.
- May occur in the context of extensive metastatic bone disease or hormone-secreting tumours.

Signs and symptoms
- Severe and intolerable symptoms—must be treated urgently.
- Pain (bone and abdominal).
- Nausea and vomiting.
- Confusion.
- Diuresis.

Management
- Involve the specialist palliative care team early.
- Treat the underlying cause, if possible (radiotherapy to multiple lytic lesions caused by leukaemia).
- Parenteral fluids.
- Diuretics.
- Bisphosphonate therapy (parenteral and po for maintenance).

Summary of palliative care emergencies
While it is true that emergencies are rare in PPM, they can cause considerable fear and suffering. To pre-empt this, those working with children with life-limiting conditions should anticipate the possibility of an emergency, recognize it early, and have a plan ready.

Management of palliative medicine emergencies always requires the involvement of tertiary services. Ideally, this should be a PPM service, but, where none is available, advice should urgently be sought from the adult palliative medicine team locally.

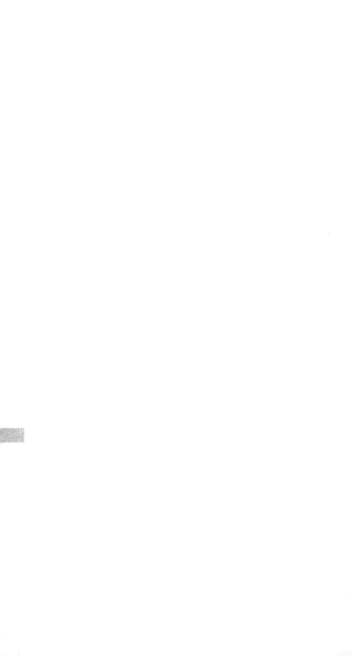

Chapter 16

Malignant diseases

Introduction

Cancer in childhood is a group of heterogeneous conditions linked largely by their pathogenesis. There are several reviews of symptoms occurring in childhood cancer. The symptoms a child will experience depend on:
- the particular diagnosis;
- its primary location;
- the pattern of spread;
- the extent and nature of prior treatment;
- its secondary consequences (e.g. bone marrow suppression).

With respect to palliative medicine, malignant diseases can be considered in three broad groups:
- haemopoietic malignancies (leukaemia and lymphoma);
- CNS tumours (usually brain);
- other solid tumours

The likelihood of needing referral for specialist palliative medicine is influenced by prognosis, as well as incidence, and therefore change as outcomes improve:
- Haemopoietic malignancies are common, but there is a good chance of cure.
- Solid tumours often carry a smaller chance of cure but are rare.
- CNS tumours are common, and, despite new therapeutic approaches, the prognosis for many remains guarded.

Central nervous system tumours
- Astrocytomas.
- Medulloblastoma.
- Ependymoma.
- Brainstem glioma.

Haemopoietic malignancies
- Acute myeloid leukaemia.
- Acute lymphoid leukaemia.
- Hodgkin's lymphoma.
- Non-Hodgkin's lymphoma.
- Chronic leukaemias (rare).

Other solid tumours
- Rhabdomyosarcoma.
- Neuroblastoma.
- Osteosarcoma.
- Ewing's sarcoma.
- Wilms' tumour.
- Other sarcomas.

Symptoms in cancer

The ten commonest symptoms experienced by children with cancer are:
• pain (92%);
• weakness (91%);
• anorexia (68%);
• weight loss (67%);
• mobility (61%);
• nausea or vomiting (59%);
• constipation (59%);
• sleep disturbance (49%);
• anxiety and depression (45%);
• dyspnoea (40%).

However, these symptoms are not experienced by all three groups equally.
Top five symptoms in non-CNS solid tumours:
• pain (98%);
• weakness (94%);
• weight loss (88%);
• anorexia (84%);
• constipation (67%).

Top five symptoms experienced by those with CNS tumours:
• weakness (93%);
• mobility problems (89%);
• pain (81%);
• difficulties with speech (76%);
• excess secretions (70%).

Top five symptoms experienced by children with haemopoietic malignancies
(leukaemia or lymphoma):
• pain (95%);
• weakness (83%);
• bleeding (66%);
• infection (59%);
• anorexia and weight loss (56%).

Despite palliative care, there is a tendency for symptoms to become more
frequent and more severe, as death approaches. This is particularly marked
for symptoms for which there are few effective interventions available,
such as:
• weakness;
• weight loss;
• swallowing, excess secretions;
• sleep disturbance.

These are also the symptoms experienced by children with CNS tumours,
making palliative care in this group particularly challenging.

The interface between oncology and palliative care

Typically, oncology patients and their families have three main fears, once it becomes clear that their battle against the disease will be lost:

- symptoms, especially pain;
- abandonment by professionals who have become familiar;
- the exact mode of death (often fears of haemorrhage, seizure, or choking).

Achieving a 'good death' for oncology patients critically depends on sensitive handling of the transition from a 'curative' to a 'palliative' phase:

- *The palliative medicine consultant and team should be introduced to the family, before curative treatment is discontinued.* Palliative management and potentially curative management can, and often should, proceed simultaneously. Families fear being abandoned by their oncology team, and it is important that there is overlap between the 'curative' and 'palliative' phases of their care, in order to allow new relationships to develop. Most tertiary paediatric oncology teams will include paediatric oncology outreach nurse specialists who may also be experienced and/or trained in paediatric palliative care and can provide important continuity.
- Involvement of new professionals at the end of life should be kept to a minimum. Discussions about what might happen at the end of life are important to families, and they must be carefully planned and sensitively paced. Continuity across home, hospital, and hospice is essential for that to happen, and involvement of multiple palliative care teams in different locations should be avoided, wherever possible.
- *'Curative' modalities often have a place in management of symptoms*, even where they cannot cure the condition. Where they might be of value in symptom management, chemotherapy, radiotherapy, and even surgery should be considered, in collaboration with the oncology team. Multiple visits for planning, fractionated doses of radiation, or frequent blood tests are to be avoided, but they are rarely required.

The role of chemotherapy once cure is no longer expected

Even once it is acknowledged that there is no prospect of cure, chemotherapy may continue to be prescribed for one or more of the following reasons:

- as part of a clinical trial;
- to 'buy time' for the child;
- at the request of family who feel that everything should be done;
- to relieve symptoms—in effect, as an adjuvant.

Although chemotherapy is often called 'palliative' in any of these situations, it is only correctly used in the last. 'Palliative' indicates that its intent is primarily to relieve symptoms.

A number of factors should inform any decision to continue chemotherapy once cure is not possible:

- Their benefit must always outweigh the burden.
- Delaying death should do more than simply prolong dying.
- It is never appropriate to prescribe chemotherapy at the request of the family, unless it is in the child's own best interest to do so.
- Many young people value the opportunity to take part in clinical trials for altruistic reasons. The principle of equipoise means it is not expected that such trials will benefit them, and this should be made clear.
- Some chemotherapy agents are relatively non-toxic and can provide significant symptom relief, if properly used (e.g. vincristine, po etoposide, po 6-mercaptopurine). In this context, chemotherapy is, in effect, acting as an adjuvant to analgesia. *This is the only correct use of the term 'palliative chemotherapy', since its purpose is to relieve symptoms without influencing disease course.*

Further reading

Goldman, A., Hewitt, M., Collins, G.S., Childs, M., and Hain, R. (2006). Symptoms in children/young people with progressive malignant disease: United Kingdom Children's Cancer Study Group/Paediatric Oncology Nurses Forum survey. *Pediatrics* 117 (6), e1179–86.

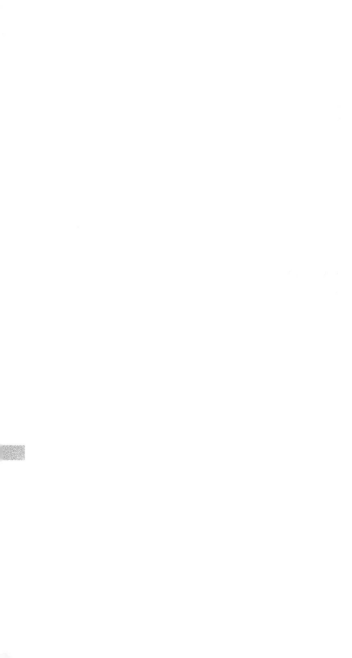

Specific non-malignant diseases

Introduction

The cross-section of life-limiting conditions affecting children is quite different from those in adults. In adult palliative care, the vast majority of work is around malignant conditions, while, in paediatric palliative care, the work is based equally on malignant and non-malignant conditions.

The number of life-limiting conditions in paediatrics is vast; the Contact a Family (CaF) directory of specific conditions and rare disorders (ℜ www.cafamily.org.uk) holds details of over 1000 different conditions. In view of this number it is almost impossible for any one doctor to know the details of all the conditions.

In the authors' opinion, it is best to have a good working knowledge of the commonest non-malignant disorders and then obtain the details of other rarer conditions, as required. In many cases of the rarer disorders, little may be known about the trajectory of the condition. In other cases, we may not even have a diagnosis and so have no idea what to expect from the illness. An empirical approach to assessment and management of illness is very effective in such situations.

There are several medical conditions that are common enough for it to be helpful to know about them in more detail. As all the conditions by definition have no cure, it is best to tackle each symptom with which the child presents individually, never forgetting that medical intervention is not the only modality open to us. The full array of the multidisciplinary team is required to effect the best holistic care. This is discussed in length in the DMD section (see Chapter 17, Duchenne muscular dystrophy, pp. 161–2), but the same principles need to be carried through with regard to other conditions.

Duchenne muscular dystrophy

DMD is the second commonest single-gene disorder in Western countries.

Genetics

- DMD is caused by a gene defect on the X chromosome at the Xp21 level. This gene produces a very large protein called dystrophin. This is present in very small amounts in normal muscle but is virtually absent or non-functional in the muscles of patients with DMD.
- Dystrophin combines with a glycoprotein to form a complex that is essential for muscle cell membrane. Disruption of the complex leads to muscle cell death.
- DMD is inherited as an X-linked recessive trait. The mutant gene is always fully penetrant.

Diagnosis

Diagnosis is confirmed with the triad of tests:
- serum creatine kinase (50–100 times normal);
- muscle biopsy;
- DNA analysis.

Clinical features

- The onset is slow, and the average age of diagnosis is 5 years (can be as late as 8–9 years).
- Early symptoms are delay in walking, tiptoeing, recurrent falls, and inability to run.
- Early signs are:
  - inability to run;
  - inability to stand on one leg (positive Trendelenburg);
  - inability to lift their head off the bed;
  - inability to rise from sitting with folded arms; the child uses his arms to climb up his thighs (Gowers' manoeuvre);
  - sliding through the examiner's hands when lifted from under the arms.
- Progression is seen over time as:
  - lumbar lordosis;
  - waddling gait;
  - equinovarus deformity from shortening of the Achilles tendon;
  - 95% of the boys become wheelchair-bound by the age of 12 years. The earlier the child becomes wheelchair-bound, the poorer the prognosis.
- Late stage signs:
  - contractures of other tendons;
  - severe kyphoscoliosis;
  - weakness of the intercostal muscles;
  - respiratory problems with hypoventilation and hypercapnia at night;
  - patients with diurnal hypercapnia will die within 9.7 months (mean value) without ventilation;
  - respiratory failure with infection is the commonest cause of death.[1]

Other organ system involvement

Although the skeletal muscle is the main tissue involved in DMD, other tissues and organs can be affected. These complications occur in only some of the children.

- Cardiac muscle:
  - involvement can lead to arrhythmia and heart failure;
  - 15% of DMD cases die of primary cardiomyopathy.
- Gastrointestinal:
  - constipation;
  - paralytic ileus;
  - gastric dilatation.
- Bladder:
  - rarely bladder paralysis.
- Vascular:
  - increased bleeding tendency noted after spinal surgery;
  - poor circulation.
- CNS:
  - lowered IQ to 80 average.
- Skeletal system (secondary to immobility, rather than disease):
  - impaired development of major bones;
  - skeletal deformity;
  - osteoporosis.

Management and prognosis for Duchenne muscular dystrophy

Management

By working as a multidisciplinary team, we can improve quality of life and increase survival. The team may consist of a number of specialties, including:

- specialist neurodisability units:
    - to supply expert advice;
    - to coordinate appropriate care.
- community and hospital paediatricians:
    - for day-to-day medical care;
    - to control symptoms.
- palliative care team:
    - to control difficult symptoms.
- dietitian:
    - to improve nutrition and weight control.
- physiotherapy:
    - to maintain ambulation as long as possible;
    - to stretch muscles and tendons, and hence reduce the severity of contractures, including teaching the parents;
    - to advise on the right forms of splints and walking aids;
    - to advise on wheelchairs, posture, and support.
- occupational therapist;
- surgeon:
    - for release of contractures;
    - to correct spinal deformity;
    - to help with the high fracture rate (up to 20%).
- cardiologist:
    - to monitor and treat all the cardiac symptoms.
- respiratory physician:
    - to monitor respiratory function and plan the best time for ventilation;
    - for treatment of respiratory infection;
    - vaccinations.
- home ventilation team:
    - to help the child and family learn about, use, and maintain the most appropriate ventilation system.
- psychologist;
- educational team;
- social services.

Prognosis

The prognosis of DMD has continued to improve over the last four decades (Table 17.1).[2] Each improvement, however, as with any incurable disease, leads to new problems that have to be faced by the patient, family, and health-care professionals.

Table 17.1 Mean age of survival over time in a patient with DMD

Decade	Mean age of survival (years)
1960s	14.3
1980s (with better medical care)	19
2000s (with ventilation)	24.3

Eagle, M., Baudouin, S.V., Chandler, C., Giddings, D.R., Bullock, R., and Bushby, K. (2002). Survival in Duchenne muscular dystrophy: improvements in life expectancy since 1967 and the impact of home nocturnal ventilation. *Neuromuscul. Disord.* 12 (10), 926–9.

Mucopolysaccharidoses

The mucopolysaccharide (MPS) illnesses are all genetic lysosomal storage conditions. MPS are now called glycosaminoglycans (GAGs). In the various conditions, there is a genetic abnormality that prevents or significantly reduces the production of specific enzymes. As a result, the body is unable to break down certain waste products. These products cannot be excreted by the body and so are stored within the lysosomes of cells throughout the body, causing damage to a wide range of tissues. The conditions caused are not apparent at birth but soon develop over time, as the storage of material increases. There is a range of conditions, but here we will discuss the three commonest types.

Mucopolysaccharidosis type 1 (Hurler's syndrome)

- There are three subsets of conditions classified as MPS type 1. Of these, Hurler's is the most severe.
- Hurler's syndrome is caused by a lack of an enzyme called lysosomal alpha-L-iduronidase.
- It is caused by a recessive gene.[3]

Clinical features

- Facial changes can be seen from 2 years of age.
- Most symptoms develop between ages 3 and 8 years.
- Growth retardation from age 3 years.
- Coarse facial features with:
  - short nose;
  - low nose bridge;
  - flat facies;
  - large head;
  - the tongue is enlarged and may stick out;
  - thick lips.
- Corneal clouding.
- Deafness.
- Musculoskeletal:
  - bent-over posture when walking;
  - scoliosis;
  - joint disease with stiffness;
  - claw hand;
  - nerve entrapment, including carpal tunnel syndrome.
- Mental retardation, dependent on severity of condition.
- Respiratory problems secondary to:
  - runny nose;
  - enlarged tonsils and adenoids;
  - chest wall deformity;
  - pressure on the diaphragm from an enlarged liver and spleen;
  - sleep apnoea;
  - recurrent chest infections.
- Cardiac problems:
  - cardiomyopathy;
  - endocardiofibroelastosis;
  - coronary heart disease;
  - aortic and mitral valve disease.
- Gastrointestinal:
  - protruding belly;
  - hepatosplenomegaly;
  - umbilical and inguinal herniae;
  - diarrhoea and constipation.

Prognosis

As there is a range of severity associated with MPS type 1, with Hurler's being the most severe, the prognosis is also variable. In the most severe cases, the child is likely to die before their teenage years; in the mildest form, the child may live into young adulthood.

Mucopolysaccharidosis type 2 (Hunter's syndrome)

- Hunter's syndrome is caused by a lack of an enzyme called iduronate sulfatase.
- It is an X-linked recessive genetic disorder.
- Originally thought of as two separate types—juvenile onset and late onset—but now thought to be a spectrum, with the two subsets just being extremes on the scale.[4]

Clinical features

As per MPS type 1, but with these additional features:
- mental retardation, dependent on severity of condition;
- aggressive behaviour.

Prognosis

In the most severe cases, the child is likely to die aged 10–20 years. In the mildest form, the patient may live up to 50 or 60 years of age.

Mucopolysaccharidosis type 3 (Sanfilippo syndrome)

- MPS type 3 is possibly the commonest type of MPS.[5]
- There are four types of Sanfilippo syndrome, characterized by four different enzyme deficiencies:
  - type A: an enzyme called heparan N-sulfatase;
  - type B: an enzyme called alpha-N-acetylglucosaminidase;
  - type C: an enzyme called acetyl-CoAlpha-glucosaminide acetyltransferase;
  - type D: an enzyme called N-acetylglucosamine 6-sulfatase.
- Clinically, all four types are the same.
- It is an autosomal recessive disorder.

Clinical features

- MPS type 3 has all the features seen in MPS types 1 and 2, but generally to a much milder level.
- Because the glycosaminoglycan that these four enzymes break down is primarily found in the CNS, the main clinical problems that are seen relate to its effect on the brain:
  - hyperactivity;
  - restlessness;
  - behavioural problems—often severe;
  - insomnia;
  - severe mental retardation;
  - unsteadiness;
  - recurrent falls;
  - loss of ambulation; some become wheelchair-bound;
  - muscle spasms;
  - dystonia;
  - seizures, both grand and petit mal;
  - difficulty swallowing;
  - chewing of fingers and clothes.

Prognosis

In the most severe cases, the child is likely to die aged 10–20 years. In the mildest form, the patient may live up to 30 years of age.

Batten's disease

- Batten's disease is part of a range of rare conditions known as neuronal ceroid lipofuscinoses (or NCLs).
- Batten's disease originally was described as the juvenile form of NCLs, but now the name appears to encompass all the various types.
- There are four main types of NCL: infantile, late infantile, juvenile, and adult.[6] Each becomes apparent and progresses differently.
- NCLs involve a build-up of an abnormal material called lipofuscin in the brain, probably due to an inability to remove or recycle protein by the brain. This same problem can occur in the eye, skin, muscle, and other tissues.
- It is an autosomal recessive disorder.

Clinical features of juvenile neuronal ceroid lipofuscinosis (Batten's disease)

- Onset between 4 and 10 years of age (mean of 5 years).
- Visual loss.
- Speech disorder.
- Epilepsy of various types.
- Myoclonus.
- Mental retardation can be very severe.
- Movement disorder.
- Behavioural problems.
- Extrapyramidal signs with unsteady gait and ataxia.
- Sleep disturbance.[7]

Prognosis

In the most severe cases, the child is likely to die in their late teens. In the milder form, the patient may live up to 30 years of age.

Spinal muscular atrophy

- Spinal muscular atrophy (SMA) is the second leading cause of neuromuscular disease.
- It is characterized by progressive muscle weakness due to degeneration of nerve cells in the anterior horn of the spinal tract and the brainstem nuclei.
- There are various subtypes, but it now appears that these are all part of a continuum of disease expression related to the genetic disorder.
- It is an autosomal recessive disorder.

Clinical features

- Onset:
  - SMA type 1, within 6 months of birth;
  - SMA type 2, 6–12 months of age;
  - SMA type 3, after 12 months of age.
- SMA type 1:
  - weakness at birth;
  - poor muscle tone;
  - muscle weakness;
  - lack of motor development;
  - mild contractures;
  - absence of tendon reflex;
  - lack of head control;
  - feeding difficulties;
  - breathing difficulties;
  - muscle fasciculations.
- SMA type 2:
  - less severe than type 1;
  - progressive weakness;
  - poor posture.
- SMA type 3:
  - least severe;
  - affects shoulder muscle and proximal muscle first;
  - progressive weakness.[8,9]

Prognosis

- Death within:
  - SMA type 1, less than 2–3 years;
  - SMA type 2, early infancy;
  - SMA type 3, within childhood.[10,11]

Trisomy 18 (Edward's syndrome)

Trisomy 18 is a genetic chromosomal condition where there is extra material within chromosome 18. It is relatively common, affecting girls three times more than boys.

Clinical features
- Low birthweight.
- Growth retardation.
- Physical appearance:
  - microcephaly;
  - micrognathia;
  - chest wall abnormality;
  - low-set ears;
  - clenched hands;
  - crossed legs.
- Neurological:
  - mental retardation;
  - seizures;
  - increased muscle tone.
- Cardiac:
  - congenital heart defects;
  - ventricular septal defect;
  - atrial septal defect;
  - patent ductus arteriosus;
  - valve defects.
- Renal:
  - polycystic kidneys;
  - hydronephrosis.
- Coloboma.
- Diastasis recti.
- Hernias:
  - umbilical;
  - inguinal.
- Undescended testes.
- Defects of hands and feet.

Prognosis
- 50% of all affected babies die within the first week of life.
- 95% of all affected babies die within 1 year.[12]

References

1. Emery, A. and Muntoni, F. (2004). *Duchenne muscular dystrophy*, third edition. Oxford University Press, Oxford.
2. Eagle, M., Baudouin, S.V., Chandler, C., Giddings, D.R., Bullock, R., and Bushby, K. (2002). Survival in Duchenne muscular dystrophy: improvements in life expectancy since 1967 and the impact of home nocturnal ventilation. *Neuromuscul. Disord.* **12** (10), 926–9.
3. National MPS Society (2008). *A guide to understanding MPS I.* Available at: ℘ http://mpssociety.org/wp-content/uploads/2011/07/booklet_MPS_I_v8.pdf.

4. National MPS Society (2008). *A guide to understanding MPS II*. Available at: ℗ http://mpssociety. org/wp-content/uploads/2011/07/booklet_MPS_II_v6.pdf.

5. National MPS Society (2008). *A guide to understanding MPS III*. Available at: ℗ http://mpssociety. org/wp-content/uploads/2011/07/booklet_MPS_III_v6.pdf.

6. Wisniewski, K.E., Zhong, N., and Philippart, M. (2001). Pheno/genotypic correlations of neuronal ceroid lipofuscinoses. *Neurology* **57** (4), 576–81.

7. Backman, M.L., Santavuori, P.R., Aberg, L.E., and Aronen, E.T. (2005). Psychiatric symptoms of children and adolescents with juvenile neuronal ceroid lipofuscinosis. *J. Intellect. Disabil. Res.* **49** (Pt 1), 25–32.

8. Moosa, A. and Dubowitz, V. (1973). Spinal muscular atrophy in childhood. Two clues to clinical diagnosis. *Arch. Dis. Child.* **48** (5), 386–8.

9. Iannaccone, S.T., Browne, R.H., Samaha, F.J., Buncher, C.R., and DCN/SMA Group (1993). Prospective study of spinal muscular atrophy before age 6 years. *Pediatr. Neurol.* **9** (3), 187–93.

10. Ignatius, J. (1994). The natural history of severe spinal muscular atrophy—further evidence for clinical subtypes. *Neuromuscul. Disord.* **4** (5–6), 527–8.

11. Russman, B.S., Buncher, C.R., White, M., Samaha, F.J., Iannaccone, S.T., and DCN/SMA Group (1996). Function changes in spinal muscular atrophy II and III. The DCN/SMA Group. *Neurology* **47** (4), 973–6.

12. Rasmussen, S.A., Wong, L.Y., Yang, Q., May, K.M., and Friedman, J.M. (2003). Population-based analyses of mortality in trisomy 13 and trisomy 18. *Pediatrics* **111** (4 Pt 1), 777–84.

Palliative care in intensive care environments

Introduction

A significant proportion of deaths in childhood, even those from life-limiting conditions, happen in an intensive care environment.[1] An effective interface between palliative care services and the neonatal or paediatric intensive care unit is important, but also presents certain specific challenges.

It is *important*, because:

- death in an intensive care environment is common, especially amongst neonates;
- it is the preferred place of care and death for many, because admissions can be long, especially on the neonatal unit, and families come to know and trust the staff there. It becomes a 'second home';
- intensive care is burdensome for the child and family, and that burden can be made easier by good symptom control;
- end-of-life decisions are often complex and require multidisciplinary working.

It is *challenging*, because:

- the intensive care environment is acutely medical. It can be difficult to find the time and space for unhurried discussions;
- there can be prolonged periods during which it is not clear whether the child will live or die, and palliative care will need to be offered, alongside invasive medical care;
- the aim of palliative care can seem to be at odds with that of intensive care if the latter is aimed solely at prolonging life;
- children are often unconscious or relatively unresponsive during admission to intensive care, so that it is not easy to assess the child's objective experience or quality of life. It is easy for the child's obvious physical needs to eclipse other aspects of her care;
- a child on intensive care is severely and acutely unwell, and it is not always easy to judge the child's usual quality of life at other times.

Intensive care in children with life-limiting conditions: two risks

Children with life-limiting conditions are doubly at risk in respect of invasive intensive care. They are vulnerable:

- *to the inappropriate introduction of invasive intensive care when, in reality, it will do the child more harm than good.* The reason is often that families have not had time to assimilate or explore the alternatives, and the medical team feel they need to 'buy time' for those discussions to happen. It can also be because the medical team making the decision is not aware that discussion has taken place, or because families are not ready to accept the reality of the life-limiting nature of their child's illness. Some families worry that by accepting death is inevitable makes it more likely that it will happen;
- *to the inappropriate withholding of intensive care when, in reality, it will do the child more good than harm.* The reason is often that decisions are made about the suitability of intensive care at some point in the child's future, which means important information about the child's needs at the time is not considered. It can also be because blanket judgements are made about the appropriateness of intensive care in certain groups

of patients (such as those with severe cerebral palsy), rather than about the needs of a specific child.

The decision as to whether intensive care should be offered to a child with a life-limiting condition can only be made for that specific child and relates to the child's condition at the moment it is considered.

Advance emergency care planning

This presents the medical team with a practical problem. In order to assess its appropriateness, the medical team needs to explore the family's understanding and expectations, and to find out what the child's usual experience of life is. However, to be sensitively handled, such discussions need to take place over many weeks for most families. There is rarely time for such explorations at the time the decision needs to be made.

When the child is well, on the other hand, there is plenty of time for discussion about the appropriateness of intensive care, but the clinical data and exact circumstances under which intensive care might be considered in the future are not known (Fig. 18.1). A robust emergency care planning (ECP) process provides a solution by serving as:

- a structure for discussing multiple possible outcomes in a timely manner, ideally well before any acute deterioration for which intensive care might be considered;
- a 'flag' to clinicians that such discussions have taken place;
- a written record of the discussions, including parents' understanding and preferences in respect of intensive care.

Child stable:
Plenty of time for discussions about ICU, but details about harm and benefit not known.

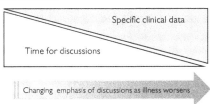

Specific clinical data

Time for discussions

Changing emphasis of discussions as illness worsens

Child acutely unwell:
Details about harm and benefit more clearly known, but little time for discussions.

Fig. 18.1 Emergency care planning process. Timely rehearsal of various possible scenarios that might lead to escalation of respiratory support is started when the child is stable and there is time for sensitive and well-paced exploration. That provides the basis for more urgent and focused discussions at the time of an acute episode, when the specific clinical data are known and a meaningful assessment can be made as to whether intensive care will do the child more good than harm.

Compassionate extubation

- *Compassionate extubation* is the name given to cessation of invasive ventilation on the grounds that it is not in the child's interests to continue.
- If it is clear or probable that continuing to ventilate a child with a life-limiting condition will cause the child more harm than good (taking into account the broadest possible definitions of 'harm' and 'good'), then it should be discontinued.
- However, as rational and necessary such an action might be, it is a decision most families find extremely difficult to hear and to participate in.
- Careful and sensitive communication is central to the palliative care team's support for the child and family.

Discussions

Timely, sensitive, and appropriately paced discussions with the child's parents are necessary for several reasons.

- The process of dialogue is an important part of the support that intensive and palliative care teams can offer families going through the death of their child.
- They will have to live with the memory of the days surrounding their child's death and of their participation in the process. One priority for palliative care is to help find 'the path of least regret'.
- The child's parents are the people most likely to know what the child is like when well, and to understand the broader potential 'quality of life' benefits for the child. Those potential benefits must inform the medical team's decision to stop ventilation.
- The medical team needs to be confident that the parents understand why ventilation is being stopped. That requires both that parents know the facts and that they understand their significance.

Note that the intensive care team does not need consent from the child's parents to stop an intervention if continuing it will probably cause more harm than good. Nevertheless, parents' preferences are an important consideration in every decision in every child, and carry authority if there is reasonable doubt about whether discontinuation is better for the child than continuing.

Inevitably, there will be times when a child's family cannot bring themselves to participate in a decision to discontinue ventilation, or disagree with the assessment of the medical team, or express a strong preference that ventilation should continue, irrespective of whether it is in the interests of the child. Under those circumstances, one or more of the following may be possible ways forward:

- careful exploration of the family's views to establish the basis for their preference (for example, it might be possible to correct a misunderstanding about the nature of the condition);
- advice from a local or national Clinical Ethics Committee;
- use of a medical mediation service;[2]
- referral to the court via legal advice.

The court will often expect or instruct that the first two are done prior to any hearing.

Parallel planning

- If discussions are left until there is no doubt that the child is dying, it will often be too late to offer families any meaningful part in them.
- If compassionate extubation is discussed at an appropriately timely moment, it will often be at a point when it remains possible that the child will not die.
- Discussions and plans therefore need to accommodate both the eventuality that the child will die and that she will recover, or at least survive for a significant period.
- That process ('We are expecting X to happen. If X happens, then we will do A. It is less likely that Y will happen. But if Y does happen, then we will do B') is described as 'parallel planning'.
- It is not uncommon to need three sets of parallel plans, but it can be difficult for families to assimilate more than that, especially as the likelihood of each diminishes.

Deciding on a place

Compassionate extubation usually takes place in the paediatric or neonatal intensive care unit (NICU). At the time it is proposed, families have often developed close relationships with the intensive care or neonatal unit staff and will express that that is where they feel 'safest'. Increasingly, children's hospices are offering their facilities, so that the tube can be removed in a less acute environment, and this is greatly welcomed by many families. If support is available, compassionate extubation can also take place in the patient's home.

Typically, parallel planning includes outlining plans for three outcomes following compassionate extubation:

- the child dies immediately in the location where extubation takes place;
- the child survives a few hours or days, requiring symptom control measures and other aspects of end-of-life care to be anticipated and easily available;
- the child unexpectedly recovers back to something approximating her baseline level of life quality.

The choice of location for compassionate extubation therefore depends on several factors, including:

- the family's own preferences;
- the practicality of transferring the child, ventilated, to a new location;
- the practicality of ensuring there is immediate access to expert symptom control, should it be needed;
- the likelihood and practicality of the child's surviving and having medical needs that necessitate transfer back to an acute paediatric unit;
- additional considerations, such as plans for the family to spend time with the child after death and arrangements for baptism or organ donation, that might make one environment more suitable than another for practical reasons.

Management of compassionate extubation, especially in an environment other than the intensive care or neonatal unit, requires careful communication and collaboration between palliative care and intensive care/neonatal teams. It should not be attempted by either team in isolation from the other.

Practicalities

As already mentioned, the key to good management of extubation is communication. The discussions that take place require a multidisciplinary approach with the child, family, and community at the centre of the decision-making process. If the extubation is to take place outside of the intensive care unit, then it is critical that these discussions should involve the community multidisciplinary team as well. The challenge for any unit is trying to bring together all the individuals that are required for this process in a short space of time. Unfortunately, time, rather than desire, often limits what can be done within an intensive care unit or when the child is discharged home or to a hospice. The key to overcoming this hurdle is pre-planning and the development of established systems and processes. When establishing such protocols, it is important to consider some of the following points.

- A full discussion should occur with the family and child, if appropriate, of the possible consequences and outcomes involved with the extubation, and an end-of-life agreement should be established, highlighting the family's and child's wishes.
- A personal resuscitation plan linked to either a do-not-resuscitate or allowed-natural-death should be written in advance of any extubation.
- A discussion should occur with the family around the anticipated symptoms such as pain and breathlessness. They should be fully informed of all the risks and benefits of the management options available.
- An honest discussion should take place with the family and child around the best place for extubation to occur, taking into account the risk, benefits, and resources, whether this is the intensive care unit, at home, or the hospice. Many families may choose to stay within the intensive care unit where they already know the team and feel secure.
- The care team around the child should be clearly identified, both in the intensive care unit but also if the child is to be transferred to the hospice or home in which case the family needs to know who the care team is in the community.
- The establishment of a key worker who can follow the child in all the different environments of hospital and community is essential.
- All children who require extubation need 24/7 access to specialist medical and nursing services. Although non-specialist services are extremely helpful, the very nature of the process of extubation requires experienced doctors and nurses.
- If a child is to be transferred to a hospice or home, then prior to discharge, an assessment needs to be made of the resources and equipment that will be required in these environments. Medical supplies should be in place. Specialist beds should be located in appropriate

areas, and specialist mattresses and other appliances should be in the home or hospice prior to discharge.
- If appropriate, a discussion should be initiated around the possibility of organ donation. If the parents wish to let them know about this, then the regional organ donation team should be involved at an early stage.
- A discussion needs to occur around any special ceremonies that the family may wish to perform either prior to or after the death of the child.
- A parallel plan of care for the child should be established, just in case the child does not die following extubation.

Transferring

Transferring a terminally ill child on a ventilator from hospital to home or hospice can be very challenging. The following issues should be considered for this process.
- A review for medications should occur prior to discharge, and non-essential medications should be withdrawn.
- A discussion should occur between the medical team and the family around the continuation of fluids and feeds. The use of iv fluids in the home or hospice may either be inappropriate or not be possible. It may be possible to continue fluids through an NG tube or a gastrostomy.
- An ambulance supporting ventilation equipment should be made available. The ambulance service should be made aware of the importance of arriving to the unit on time and transferring the child to the receiving unit on time.
- A clear plan needs to have been developed in advance of what course of action would need to be taken, should the child die en route in the ambulance.
- For a home transfer, the transferring team should be made fully aware of the practicalities of the environment into which they will be moving the child. This includes issues around lifts and access through doors and rooms.
- When the child arrives at the hospice or home, the receiving team should be in attendance. It should be made clear at the onset of the different roles of the two teams. This should include which equipment will be taken back to the intensive care unit and which is to remain with the child. There should also be a clear understanding about when extubation will actually take place and who will conduct the extubation itself.
- The transferring team should have quick and easy transport back to the unit for the staff and all equipment.

Symptom management/anticipation

Symptom management is a process that should have been occurring throughout the child's journey. However, extubation itself carries its own challenges, in terms of drug management and ethics. The ethics issues are discussed later (see ➲ Chapter 3, Ethics). The following issues should be considered, in terms of management.

- The child should be discharged with a supply of the medications that they are taking. A minimum of a 2-day supply for a hospice and 7-day supply for a home discharge is required.
- A supply of anticipatory medicines for pain and symptom management should be immediately available either at the hospice or in the home.
- Specialist doctors from the intensive care unit, paediatric palliative consultants, or GPs with special interest in PPM need to be in attendance during all extubations, so that they can immediately manage any symptoms that may arise.
- It is often helpful to preload a child with medication prior to extubation and to have anticipatory drugs already drawn up when the extubation itself does occur.
- The dose of benzodiazepine should be appropriate for the management of dyspnoea (e.g. midazolam 0.05mg/kg sc or buccally prn every 30–60min).
- The dose of opioid should be appropriate for management of dyspnoea (50% of the analgesic dose).
- A dose of steroids may be helpful, as it is thought that the child may experience noisy breathing from laryngeal oedema.
- We do not use medication that can cause muscle paralysis.
- All children should have 24/7 access to specialist medical and nursing support.

After death
Many of the issues to consider after the death of a child are covered in various chapters within this book. Some of the key issues to consider are:
- the need to provide emotional and spiritual support for the parents after the death of their child;
- the importance of considering the emotional and spiritual needs of siblings and grandparents;
- all child deaths in England and Wales have to be reported to the coroner. The coroner will then decide whether this is a case he wishes to investigate or if he is happy to authorize the issue of a death certificate;
- all deaths in England and Wales have to be reported to the child death review panel who will investigate the deaths to see if there are any learning points from the case;
- the issues around post-mortems can be very difficult for the family. Sometimes a post-mortem may be mandatory, e.g. post-mortems requested by the coroner. At other times, a post-mortem may be requested by the family themselves or the hospital physicians to help with improving diagnosis and for research purposes. All these issues should have been discussed at the very start of the process;
- if the parents had consented to organ donation prior to the child's death, then the regional organ donation team will guide the family through the processes involved with donation;
- the issuing of death certificates is straightforward, unless the child had died while in transit from the hospital to home or the hospice. The discussions prior to the extubation should have provided the documentation on who would be responsible for issuing the certificate under these circumstances.

'Failure to die' and the need to care for the unstable child

One of the great difficulties within PPM is predicting the prognosis of any child who is terminal. It is well recognized that, after extubation, many children will continue to breathe spontaneously and may do so for hours, days, weeks, months, or years. It is therefore critical that, in all cases of compassionate extubation, a parallel plan should be made for these circumstances. The parallel plan should consider:

- when to re-instigate fluids and feeds;
- when to re-instigate medication that was previously withdrawn;
- which paediatrician will continue to take the role of lead paediatrician for the care of the child. In many circumstances, this will not be the intensive care or palliative care consultant but may be a community paediatrician;
- if a child is in the hospital or hospice, then a clear plan of discharge back into the community should be available;
- additional nursing and social support services may be required for the child to continue to live at home;
- the child may continue to need specialist paediatric palliative medical and nursing support;
- the family may need additional emotional and spiritual support, after having gone through the emotional experience of thinking their child would die and then seeing them live for a little while longer.

Ethics

Why ventilate children with life-limiting conditions?

Intensive care, and invasive ventilation in particular, is uncomfortable and traumatic. It might be argued that it has no place in the management of a child with a life-limiting condition, because their function is essentially to keep a patient alive while she recovers from a reversible illness. If the illness is not reversible, it might be argued the harms cannot be justified.

Some children with life-limiting conditions will nevertheless require invasive intensive care interventions, for example, because:

- it is not always clear that a child's condition is life-limiting at the time intensive care is instituted (for example, hypoxic–ischaemic brain injury at birth);
- individual episodes might be reversible. A child might recover her baseline health and well-being, even if an acute episode is in the context of a condition that will eventually kill her;
- the alternative is worse (for example, if the family needs time for sensitive and well-paced discussions about end-of-life care).

All three are illustrations of a situation in which the probable benefits of invasive ventilation, taken in the broadest possible sense, justify its certain harms.

Should disability make a difference?

Families are often anxious that appropriate intensive care will be withheld or withdrawn from their child on the basis that she has a life-limiting condition, because they worry that medical teams underestimate, or even fail to take account altogether of, the child's capacity to enjoy her life despite her disability.

That fear can be exacerbated by any perception that a unit is operating a 'triage' system, in which greater priority for resources is given to children whose underlying condition is curable.

In the context of a luxurious health-care system (i.e. one, like the National Health Service (NHS), that provides its users with more than is strictly necessary), any such triage would be ethically problematic. Nevertheless, it would be equally unfair to claim that the nature of a child's underlying condition was of no relevance to how they should be treated in the most ethically acceptable way. The certain harms of intensive care must be set against the probable benefits. Those benefits are directly dependent on the child's abilities.

It is always true that intensive care should only continue while it will probably offer the individual child more benefit than harm. To that extent, a child's disability makes no difference. An able child is not inherently more entitled to intensive care than a child with a disability.

But the specific goods and harms that intensive care might do are related to the extent and nature of an individual child's disability and, for that reason, are relevant to the decision to discontinue ventilation through compassionate extubation.

Symptoms during compassionate extubation

- Extubation carries a risk of symptoms of dyspnoea, as the child gasps for breath.
- A concern for clinicians is that interventions, such as opioids and benzodiazepines, that might relieve dyspnoea will reduce respiratory effort that might otherwise allow the child to survive.
- If they are properly prescribed, that risk is small, because the dose required to relieve an unpleasant sense of breathlessness is much less than a dose that would abolish respiratory effort.
- There is no place in the management of symptoms during compassionate extubation for drugs that cause muscle paralysis.
  - Although such drugs abolish the *appearance* of respiratory distress, they do not abolish the child's experience of it.
  - On the contrary, they potentially amplify that distress by preventing the child's ability to gasp and by making it impossible for carers to recognize and treat the child's distress.
  - Furthermore, they remove any chance that the child will survive, meaning that death is from drug poisoning, rather than from the underlying condition.

Review of resources

The idea of compassionate extubation is not new to anyone who has worked within the intensive care units of hospitals.[3] However, the fact that compassionate extubation can be improved by good communication and processes has developed interest over the last decade.[4] In addition, with improvements in technology and increased palliative medicine experience, it is becoming increasingly recognized that this can be done from hospices or, in fact, at home.[5-8] Together for Short Lives, through its 2011 document *Care pathway to support extubation within children's palliative care network*,[9] has produced a document that provides all the resources necessary to begin the process of developing protocols and pathways to allow compassionate extubation.

Summary of palliative care in intensive care environments

- At first sight, it seems that intensive care and palliative care are at opposite ends of the care spectrum. The paediatric intensive care unit (PICU) and NICU rely on high-tech invasive interventions and analysis of physiological parameters, measured using precise numerical data. In palliative care, interventions are typically few and basic, and clinical decisions are typically characterized by discussion, ambiguity, and uncertainty.
- But families should not have to see intensive and palliative care as alternative to one another. Intensive care environments are the most likely clinical settings for good end-of-life care to be needed. Families live for weeks at a time, knowing that death and recovery are both quite likely outcomes and having to adjust simultaneously to the possibility of both of them. Families expect doctors to prioritize their child's comfort in the present at the very same time as optimizing the chances of their recovery in the future. And they are right to expect that. Intensive and palliative care are orientated towards the same goal—enabling a child to enjoy the best possible quality of life for as long as possible.
- Those goals are, in reality, rarely in conflict. Intensive care that is proportionate and compassionately delivered is a form of palliative care, if it enables a child to enjoy more of a life that has quality. Similarly, intensive care can be made tolerable by the sort of attention to physical, emotional, and existential aspects of care that constitutes good palliative medicine.

But in practice, the ethos of PICUs or NICUs often seem in tension with that of palliative care. Intensive care environments may represent the single most important interface with palliative care in paediatrics. They also offer perhaps the greatest challenge.

References

1. Bluebond-Langner, M., Beecham, E., Candy, B., Langner, R., and Jones, L. (2013). Preferred place of death for children and young people with life-limiting and life-threatening conditions: a systematic review of the literature and recommendations for future inquiry and policy. *Palliat. Med.* **27** (8), 705–13.

2. Forbat, L., Teuten, B., and Barclay, S. (2015). Conflict escalation in paediatric services: findings from a qualitative study. *Arch. Dis. Child* **100** (8), 769–73.

3. Janvier, A., Meadow, W., Leuthner, S.R., et al. (2011). Whom are we comforting? An analysis of comfort medications delivered to dying neonates. *J. Pediatr.* **159** (2), 206–10.

4. Mitchell, S., Plunkett, A., and Dale, J. (2014). Use of formal advance care planning documents: a national survey of UK Paediatric Intensive Care Units. *Arch. Dis. Child* **99** (4), 327–30.

5. Laddie, J., Craig, F., Brierley, J., Kelly, P., and Bluebond-Langner, M. (2014). Withdrawal of ventilatory support outside the intensive care unit: guidance for practice. *Arch. Dis. Child* **99** (9), 812–16.

6. Garcia-Salido, A., Monleón-Luque, M., Barceló-Escario, M., Del Rincón-Fernández, C., Catá-Del Palacio, E., and Martino-Alba, R. (2014). [Withdrawal of assisted ventilation in the home: making decisions in paediatric palliative care]. *An. Pediatr. (Barc.)* **80** (3), 181–3.

7. E. C. Simpson, and Penrose, C.V. (2011). Compassionate extubation in children at hospice and home. *Int. J. Palliat. Nurs.* **17** (4), 164–9.

8. Zwerdling, T., Hamann, K.C., and Kon, A.A. (2006). Home pediatric compassionate extubation: bridging intensive and palliative care. *Am. J. Hosp. Palliat. Care* **23** (3), 224–8.

9. ACT (Association for Children's Palliative Care) (2011). *A care pathway to support extubation within a children's palliative care framework.* ACT, Bristol.

Chapter 19

Practicalities around time of death

Introduction

There are different types of paediatric death:
1. sudden unexpected death in a normal child;
2. a child with a life-limiting condition who dies unexpectedly;
3. a child with a life-limiting condition who has an expected death.

For the purpose of this chapter, we will be discussing points 2 and 3, but health-care professionals dealing with a situation in point 1 may still find much of the information useful.

In helping children to have a 'good death', it is vitally important to understand the practical issues around death. Parents often have little or no understanding of this and will look to the health-care professional for guidance. When done well, the parents are left unaware of the complexities involved. However, when done badly, the parents can be left feeling very upset.

The legal aspects to death in this chapter pertain to UK law.[1] Readers in other countries should make themselves familiar with the law of the country in which they are practising.

Predictors of death

Predicting the time of death for a child is notoriously difficult.[2] Experience has taught us that we are frequently having to tell parents that their child is about to die, only for the child to recover and be discharged home. Sadly, this is only temporary, and the child then presents again days, weeks, or months later. This emotional rollercoaster is very draining for the parents. We often recommend to the parents that they should take each day as it comes.

In some situations, we can, as health-care professionals, anticipate that a child's condition may continue to deteriorate on to death:
- certain malignancies such as brain tumours;
- malignancies where all forms of treatment have failed, and disease progression is seen as rapid;
- when specific organ failure is occurring such as liver or renal failure, and the rate is documented as progressive;
- a child starts to have increasingly prolonged periods of sleep apnoea;
- seizure frequency and intensity continue to increase to a level where the seizures and the treatment for them begin to lead to secondary infection or respiratory suppression;
- Cheyne–Stokes breathing occurs.

Before death

When we know that death is inevitable, certain actions can be taken to help the situation.

- Check with the parents regarding their wishes (this may take many conversations).
- Check with the child if they are able to communicate.
- Follow any advanced directive protocol (individual or regional).
- All unnecessary drugs should be stopped.
- All unnecessary tubes, lines, and monitors should be removed.
- A personal resuscitation plan (PRP) should be discussed and recorded.
- In the hospice, clear instructions regarding the parents' wishes should be documented in the notes.
- At home, the ambulance service should be notified not to resuscitate, and clear instructions to the out-of-hours services should be logged on to their computer system.
- Allow family and friends unlimited access to the child (subject to the child and parents not being overwhelmed).
- Call whichever religious leader the family request.
- Allow the family to approach the death of their child in the way they think best (some children have passed away listening to their favourite music, having early birthday or Christmas parties, or even dying peacefully in their bed but outside in the garden).

Certifying and registering a death

When a child dies, the parents will often turn to the health-care professional for confirmation of death.

- At this stage, the doctor should be called.
- Suitably trained nurses can 'verify' death, but only doctors may 'certify' death for legal purposes.
- To verify/certify death, check the following:
  - feel for the carotid or femoral pulse for 1 full minute;
  - listen for breath sounds, and observe the rise and fall of the chest for 1 full minute;
  - examine the eyes for pupil reaction using a torch. Pupils should be fixed and dilated.
- Inform the family/next of kin that death has taken place.

At this stage, the doctor needs to ascertain as to whether the death needs to be referred to the coroner immediately, e.g. unexpected or suspicious deaths, or routinely. All children's deaths have to be reported to the coroner by law (see ➲ Coroner, p. 193). Routine deaths are reported during normal working hours, and the coroner will then decide if they wish to look further into the case.

If the death was expected and not expected to become a coroner's case, then:

- the doctor should issue a death certificate (Box 19.1);
- the family can call their funeral director;
- the funeral director will give detailed information to the family regarding the processes involved for the funeral;
- the body can be kept at home (see ➲ Looking after the body, p. 192) or transferred to the funeral director's offices;
- within a hospice, the body can be moved to the 'special room';
- the child's key worker should arrange for all the health-care professionals involved with the child to be notified of the death.

Registrar of births and deaths

- All deaths have to be registered by the registrar of births and deaths.
- It is best to phone and book a special appointment to save the family the distress of attending when other ceremonies may be going on.
- The family must present the death certificate to the registrar where the child died within 5 days of the child's death.
- The registrar will then issue the 'certificate for disposal'. This will allow the funeral directors to proceed with the funeral arrangements.

Box 19.1 Issuing a death certificate

- Best practice is that the doctor completing the death certificate should have seen the child in the last 14 days of life. If this has not been practical, the doctor can usually still issue a certificate following discussion with the coroner.
- Verification and certification of death are not the same (see this section).

Cremation

Cremation is becoming increasingly popular in the UK (70% of all registered deaths in 2001). Many religions have differing rules regarding cremation (see ➔ Chapter 20), and, in some faiths, this can also be dependent on the age of the child.

Certain legal rules have to be followed to allow cremation.

- The family must apply for cremation with Form 1.
- Then the doctor who completed the death certificate must complete Form 4.
  1. The doctor must see the body after death.
  2. He or she should have looked after the child for more than 24h.
  3. He or she should have seen the child within 14 days.
- If points 2 and 3 cannot be met, then the doctor must discuss the case with the coroner and obtain permission that 'no further action is required'.
- The doctor who completed Form 4 must then bring in another medical practitioner of at least 5 years' postgraduate registration, who has neither attended nor been otherwise concerned with the care or treatment of the child and who is not a relative or partner of the medical practitioner signing Form 4.
- The second doctor then must examine the child's body and complete Form 5. He must also speak to either another doctor, nurse, or member of the family to ensure that they have no concerns regarding the cause of death. The family should be pre-warned about this, as they may find it distressing to have an unknown doctor asking them questions and examining their child. Many religions also have rules about who can touch the child after death.
- Finally, the 'authority to cremate' (Form 10) is signed by the medical referee for the crematorium.
- If the coroner has issued the death certificate, then Forms 4 and 5 are not required.

Transporting the body

Irrespective of legal niceties, most police forces feel they have an obligation to treat with suspicion the discovery of any dead child in an unusual context. For this reason, funeral directors should always be the ones to transport a child's body.

Although some families may wish to transport the body home or to the hospice by car, this should be discouraged. Firstly, the driver may be emotionally upset and unsafe to drive the car. Secondly, if there is a crash, and the police find a dead child in the car, it is likely to cause serious legal problems. If this is very important to a family, the local police should be involved in the discussions from the outset.

Organ/tissue donation

- Organ donation should be considered and discussed with families, when appropriate.
- Organ donation can give the family a sense of positivity and the feeling that something good might come out of their personal tragedy.
- Organs can only be donated if they are healthy. Unfortunately, due to the nature of many of the paediatric deaths seen in life-limited disorders, actual donation from this group is low.
- Cases where organ donation is not allowed include:
  - malignancy (except primary brain tumours);
  - genetic and neurodegenerative disorders affecting multiple organs;
  - human immunodeficiency virus (HIV);
  - viral hepatitis;
  - major sepsis.
- Most organ donations come from trauma cases via PICUs.
- Tissue donation for diagnosis or research purposes can be very helpful for the family and often give them a sense of helping another child in a similar position.
- Although many religions have their own beliefs around organ and tissue donation, it is best not to prejudge but to actually ask the family what their wishes are directly.

Post-mortem

Post-mortem may be requested for a number of reasons:
- looking at the effects of the illness on specific parts of the body;
- getting biopsies from tissue that would not otherwise be available, e.g. brain tissue;
- trying to obtain information to confirm the diagnosis;
- by instruction of the coroner (special rules apply).

In all these situations (subject to religious constraint), parents may well give permission for a post-mortem. This is particularly so if they feel it may help other children with similar conditions or when a genetic diagnosis may have an influence on future pregnancies.

It is important to remember that parents will see 'tissue' or 'pathology' samples or 'organs' differently from the medical view. To them, these are parts of their child. This is particularly true of some organs such as the heart and brain.
- It is always important to reassure the parents that:
  - the procedure is surgical and the child would be sutured up afterwards;
  - all organs and tissue would be replaced, unless specific consent is given to retain certain tissues or organs;
  - dependent on the circumstances, the post-mortem can be limited to certain areas, tissues, or organs;
  - the child's face would not be damaged;
  - the child's body would be respected throughout the process;
  - the doctors will arrange to talk to the parents afterwards about any of the findings if the parents so wish.

Looking after the body

In the home
- Under normal circumstances, a child's body can be kept in the home for up to 2–3 days.
- In warmer weather, this time frame is reduced.
- It would be prudent to put a waterproof cover on the child's bed.
- Cotton wool can be put as a plug into the anus.
- It is important that any room used in the family's house has free flow of air.
- Home air conditioning units can be used.
- Air fresheners can be helpful.
- It is important to keep all insects out of the room.
- For longer periods of time, the funeral directors can take the child's body to their offices and embalm it, and then return it back within several hours.

At the hospice
- Most children's hospices have 'special rooms'.
- These look like, and are the size of, normal bedrooms but have an industrial-level refrigeration unit attached to allow the room to cool down.
- The child's body can be kept longer, without the need for embalming.
- Parents can grieve, while having the benefits of the internal bereavement support structures and resources of the hospice.
- The parents can access the child's body at any time. Parents often wish to see the child in the evening or at night.
- The bereavement support team can help:
  - the families adjust to the loss of the child;
  - if required with washing, dressing, and putting the child into the coffin;
  - to collect items for a memory box;
  - the siblings if they wish to see the child's body;
  - with follow-up support for the whole family for whatever length of time is required.
- The child can be taken straight from the 'special room' to the funeral.

At the hospital
- The child's body can be stored in the hospital mortuary.
- All hospitals have a chapel of rest where family and friends can view the body.

At the funeral director's
- The child's body can be stored in the funeral director's mortuary.
- All funeral directors have a chapel of rest where family and friends can view the body.
- The funeral director's offices are often near the family's home.

Coroner

The coroner is either a lawyer or doctor (often both) who is responsible for investigating unnatural or sudden deaths of which the cause is unknown.

The coroner's authority is conducted through the police force. This is important, as families, unless pre-warned, may become distressed at seeing police cars outside their house or police officers inside their homes.

The coroner needs to be informed of all children's deaths. He is particularly interested in cases:

- where the deceased was not attended during his last illness by a registered medical practitioner;
- if the registrar has been unable to obtain a duly completed certificate of the cause of death, or where it appears to the registrar, from the particulars contained in such certificate or otherwise, that the deceased was not seen by the certifying medical practitioner *either* after death *or* within 14 days;
- where the cause of death appears to be unknown;
- if the registrar has reason to believe that the death was unnatural or caused by violence or neglect, or by abortion, or was attended by suspicious circumstance;
- where it appears to the registrar that the death occurred during an operation or before recovery from the effects of an anaesthetic;
- where it appears to the registrar, from the contents of any medical certificate, that the death was due to industrial disease or industrial poisoning;
- if the deceased had an operation in the preceding 12 months that might be related to the cause of death.

If a doctor suspects that the death was suspicious in any way, then the following needs to occur.

- The doctor calls the coroner's office.
- The doctor should inform the parents.
- The family cannot refuse to have the coroner involved.
- Nothing should be touched around the child; the body should not be moved.
- No tubes, lines, or instruments can be removed without prior discussion with the coroner.
- The coroner's officers will take details from all the health-care professionals and the family.
- The coroner's officers will arrange for the child's body to be transferred by funeral directors to an approved hospital for a post-mortem.

Subsequently, the coroner will obtain information from all the sources. He or she has three options.

1. If the child's doctor can provide a legal death certificate, then the coroner can approve the certificate to the registrar.
2. If the child's doctor cannot provide a legal death certificate, then the coroner can authorize a post-mortem (the family cannot refuse this). From the post mortem, the coroner can issue a death certificate.
3. If the death falls into certain categories, then the coroner can call an inquest, with or without a jury. The body is often released for burial or cremation, before the inquest takes place.

Child Death Overview Panel

It is mandatory to report all children's deaths to the Child Death Overview Panel (CDOP).

The CDOP is a statutory group of the Local Safeguarding Children Board under Section 14(2) of the Children Act 2004.[3] They are responsible for:
- collecting and analysing information about each death, with a view to identifying:
  - any case giving rise to the need for a review mentioned in regulation 5(1)(e);
  - any matters of concern affecting the safety and welfare of children in the area of the authority;
  - any wider public health or safety concerns arising from a particular death or from a pattern of deaths in that area; and
- putting in place procedures for ensuring that there is a coordinated response by the authority, their Board partners, and other relevant persons to an unexpected death.

References

1. Smale, D.A. (2002). *Law of burial, cremation and exhumation*, seventh edition. Shaw and Sons, Crayford.
2. Brook, L. and Hain, R. (2008). Predicting death in children. *Arch. Dis. Child.* **93** (12), 1067–70.
3. Children Act 2004. Available at: http://www.legislation.gov.uk/ukpga/2004/31/contents.

Chapter 20

Religion and ritual

Introduction

Religion and ritual have featured in human society for many thousands of years. The fact that they have survived and are still embraced by cultures across the world exemplifies their use and the benefits to human kind. Over time, many rituals have changed and been modified, as society develops and integrates, with migration playing its part. This can lead to different rituals within different cultures of the same religion. When this happens, the danger of stereotyping should always be borne in mind.

The complexity of the rituals of different religions and their diversity can seem overwhelming at times, but interestingly all religions appear to follow many similar themes, particularly surrounding death. Even though each culture has its own approach to death, in almost all faiths, death is seen as a time of transition.

The rituals surrounding death can allow a release of emotions with support from the community around the bereaved. Pathological grief is sometimes seen when this support is not available, particularly for immigrants who do not have local cultural links.

Many individual factors, such as age, gender, and cause of death of the child, can influence how the family responds in terms of the rituals they adopt. Even if these may appear to contrast strongly with our own beliefs, it is important to respect the family's wishes and support them appropriately. This view should also encompass respecting their individual ritual specialist.

With the changes occurring within society, it is important to recognize that different generations may behave differently in response to death within the same culture. Also, people are not necessarily familiar with their own religious ritual around death.

Finally, we need to recognize that even individuals who say they do not belong to a particular religion or faith may hold very strong ethical and spiritual beliefs. It is equally important to understand these beliefs and support the individual appropriately.

Christianity

- Christians believe that there is only one God and that Jesus Christ is the 'Son of God' who was sent to save mankind.
- Their religious beliefs stem from events recorded in the Bible.
- They believe that those who repent of their sins and turn to Jesus Christ will be forgiven and will join him in heaven after death.
- Over time, many subgroups have appeared, but the largest group worldwide is represented by Catholics. There is such great variation in traditions that it is important to check with each family regarding their individual denomination.

Symbols and spiritual advisers

- The symbol is the cross of Christ.
- Spiritual advisors vary, depending on the particular denomination or sect. They range from priests or vicars to religious elders.

Specific issues

- Some faiths may fast for Lent.
- There are normally no objections to organ donations.
- There are many sects with individual laws such as the restriction of Jehovah's Witnesses regarding blood transfusion.

Before and after death for Catholics (variations for other denominations)

- A priest can be called to anoint the dying child and provide spiritual support to the child and family.
- Privacy should be provided.
- Babies can be baptized.
- Mass is part of the funeral service.
- Non-Catholics cannot take communion.

Visiting the home or church

There are no special limitations or rules beyond common courtesies.

Funeral

- The body can be buried or cremated.
- The open coffin can be displayed in the church on the night before the burial, and a vigil kept.
- The common structure of the funeral service is:
  - the bidding;
  - the word;
  - prayer;
  - the commendation;
  - the committal.

Many other Christian groups have simpler versions of this.

Anniversary of death

There are no special rules, but many families find it helpful to attend a remembrance service or follow a specific ritual on special dates or anniversaries.

Islam

- Islam is one of the most commonly held religions worldwide, and the second largest in the UK.
- Muslims believe that there is only one God (Allah) and that Muhammad (peace be on him) was the last of a line of prophets.
- The holy book is called the Qur'an.
- Muslims believe in life after death in the form of resurrection at the day of judgement. Death is predetermined by God, and death and suffering are part of God's plan.
- There are five pillars to the faith:
  - belief in one God;
  - daily prayers;
  - fasting during Ramadan;
  - giving alms (2.5% of income);
  - pilgrimage to Makkah (Hajj).

Symbols and spiritual advisers

- Symbols are the crescent moon and star.
- Islam has no ordained priesthood. Each community has its own local spiritual leader, the 'Imam', who performs religious duties, including teaching.

Specific issues

- The extended family is important, and decisions often require the approval of the head of the family (not always the father of the child).
- Young children are not expected to fast during Ramadan. From the age of 7 years, the children may fast for a few specific days with their parents. From the age of 12 years, they will often fast for the full month.
- Any adult or child who is ill can be excused from fasting.
- Muslims believe in life after death, and, as such, it is important to continue in a form that makes the preservation of the body essential. Thus, they do not agree with organ donation and accept post-mortem examinations only if legally required.
- Pork and pork products are prohibited, as is the meat of other animals that is not 'halal' (killed according to Islamic law).

Before and after death

- Before death, family members may sit with the child and read verses from the Qur'an.
- The child should face Makkah.
- The Declaration of faith (Shahada) is said.
- Holy water may be placed in the child's mouth.
- Just before death, a family member may whisper into the child's ear the call to prayer.
- After death:
  - the child is laid flat;
  - their face is pointed towards Makkah;
  - their feet are put together;
  - their arms to the side;

- their eyes closed;
- their chin is wrapped in cloth to prevent mouth opening;
- their body is washed by same-sex members of the family;
- their body is shrouded in white linen without any religious emblems.
- The body should not be touched by non-Muslims.
- Do not remove any religious objects or threads.
- Children are not permitted to attend rituals. They are discouraged from asking questions and are expected to forget death as soon as possible.

Visiting the home or mosque
- There is a very strict social etiquette within the community.
  - Men and women normally worship separately—men at the mosque and women at home.
  - Men and women do not normally shake hands.
  - Women should dress modestly.
- If visiting the mosque, there may be separate entrances for men and women. Men cover their heads, and women are expected to cover their heads, arms, and legs.
- Muslim families adopt an open house to those people paying their respects after a child's death.
  - Shoes should be removed when entering the home.
  - Red should not be worn.

Funeral
- The child should be buried within 24h by men.
- The grave is aligned, so that the child's face can be turned sideways to face Makkah.
- Women and children do not attend the burial but can attend the funeral ceremony at the mosque.
- Flowers are normally accepted.
- After burial, prayers are said at the mosque or home, and then the family will eat.
- There is great variation in expression of grief. Some sects lament loudly; others maintain serene stoicism.
- On the 3rd, 7th, and 40th day after the death, the men will gather to say prayers.
- Mourning normally lasts 3 days, with the family staying indoors; then for up to 40 days, the grave can be visited, and alms given to the poor.

Anniversary of death
- On the first anniversary, a ceremony is held, prayers said, and food served. A stone may be placed on the grave.

Hinduism

- Hinduism is the oldest religion in the world, and the third largest in the UK.
- Hindus believe in a Supreme Spirit that represents an Ultimate Reality.
- Because it is not possible for humans to comprehend this Supreme Spirit, they worship the different aspects of the universe in which it resides. These aspects are personalized as gods and deities.
- The three key gods are:
  - Brahma the Creator;
  - Vishnu the Preserver;
  - Shiva the Destroyer.
- Hindus believe in reincarnation based on the actions in one's life (karma).

Symbols and spiritual advisers

- The symbol Om is regarded as sacred.
- Hindus have many sacred texts. The oldest are the Vedas.
- The Bhagavad-Gita is the most widely read.
- Hindu priests (pandits) perform holy rites.

Specific issues

- Hindus have very strong extended family ties.
- Families often have small shrines within the home.
- There are no religious objections to organ donation or post-mortem examination.
- Many Hindus are vegetarian, and almost all do not eat beef. The right hand is used for eating, and the left hand is used for personal hygiene.

Before and after death

- Before death, family members may sit with the child and read prayers.
- Holy water from the Ganges and the sacred Tulsi leaf may be placed in the child's mouth.
- A child should die while hearing the name of God.
- At the time of death, the family may grieve loudly.
- After death:
  - the child is laid flat, sometimes lifted to the floor;
  - the body is washed by the family;
  - the body is wrapped in a white shroud or white clothes;
  - the body is placed in a coffin and a coin, gold piece, or Tulsi leaf is placed in their mouth;
  - the face is left uncovered;
  - the body is anointed and garlanded with flowers.
- The body should be touched as little as possible.
- Do not remove any religious objects or threads.

Visiting the home or temple

- Normal social courtesies apply.
- Shoes should be removed when entering the home.
- If entering a room with a shrine in the house, then shoes should be removed, and women should cover their heads.
- In the temple, everyone must remove shoes, and women should cover their heads.
- People can pray individually or as a congregation.

Funeral

- Hindus are cremated, although young babies may be buried.
- The child should be cremated within 24h.
- Flowers are accepted.
- The body is normally taken home first, and then by the family to the temple before going to the crematorium.
- The mourners walk around the body in an anticlockwise direction to symbolize the unwinding of the thread of life.
- The ashes are scattered in running water.
- Mourning normally lasts for 10 days (but can last up to 40 days), during which time the family wear white.
- On the 11th or 13th day, a final ceremony is held.
- Money is given to charity.

Anniversary of death

- On anniversaries, a ceremony is held, prayers said, and food served.
- The family may not attend other religious festivals in the first year.

Sikhism

- Sikhism is one of the newest religions in the world, and the fourth largest in the UK.
- Sikhs believe in one God.
- They believe in equality of all people and that life should involve work, worship, and charity.
- Sikhism rejects ritual.
- They believe in reincarnation and karma.
- The religion was founded in the fifteenth century by Guru Nanak.
- The Sikh holy book is the Guru Granth Sahib.

Symbols and spiritual advisers

- The Sikh symbol is the khanda.
  - There are five religious symbols (known as the '5 Ks') of great importance to Sikhs:
  1. kesh: uncut hair;
  2. kangha: comb;
  3. karra: ridged bangle worn on the right wrist;
  4. kacha: a pair of shorts;
  5. kirpaan: a short sword.
- Sikhs have no specific religious hierarchy, but each temple has a group of elders.

Specific issues

- There are no religious objections to organ donation or post-mortem examinations.
- Many Sikhs are vegetarian, and almost all those who eat meat will not eat beef. The right hand is used for eating, and the left for personal hygiene.

Before and after death

- Before death, family members may sit with the child and read prayers.
- Holy water or Amrit may be placed in the child's mouth.
- A child should die while hearing the name of God, Waheguru (wonderful Lord), being recited.
- Generally, Sikhs are happy for non-Sikhs to tend the body.
- After death:
  - the body is washed and dressed by the same-sex members of the family;
  - the body is covered in a white sheet;
  - many parents would wish for their child to wear the '5 Ks', and an older child a turban;
  - the body is placed in a coffin, and gifts of dried fruit, clothes, or money may be put in.
- Do not remove any religious objects or threads.

Visiting the home or temple (Gurudwara)

- Normal social courtesies apply.
- Shoes should be removed when entering the home.
- In the temple, everyone must remove shoes, and both men and women should cover their heads.
- On entering the prayer room, all worshippers bow their heads in front of the Guru Granth Sahib.

Funeral

- Sikhs are cremated, although young babies may be buried.
- The child should be cremated within 24h.
- Flowers are accepted.
- The body is normally taken home first, and then to the Gurudwara before going to the crematorium.
- The ashes are scattered in running water.
- Mourning normally lasts for 10 days, during which time the family wear white.
- During this time, there is normally a complete reading of the Guru Granth Sahib.
- Money is given to charity.

Anniversary of death

There are no special rules, but many families find it helpful to attend a remembrance service or follow a specific ritual on special dates or anniversaries.

Judaism

- Judaism is one of the oldest monotheistic religions of the world.
- Jews believe in one God with whom they have a covenant.
- Judaism has many texts, but the main one is the Torah.
- Orthodox Jews follow the traditional interpretation of the will of God in the Torah.
- Progressive Jews follow a modern interpretation of the ancient laws.
- Two of the Jewish commandments are to honour the dead and comfort the mourners.

Symbols and spiritual advisers

- The Jewish symbol is the Star of David.
- Spiritual leaders are known as Rabbis.

Specific issues

- There are many variations in Jewish custom at the time of death.
- Hasidic Jews do not shake hands with women and prefer not to look at, or speak with, them.
- Orthodox Jews require kosher food (with certain rituals attached).
- They also do not allow organ donation, with the exception of the cornea.
- All Jews decline post-mortem examinations, unless legally required.

Before and after death

- Before death, the rabbi should be called to recite specific prayers.
- At the point of death, no one should leave the room.
- Generally, only the family should handle the body; non-Jews should wear gloves.
- After death:
  - the body is tended by family of the same sex;
  - the body is covered in a sheet;
  - eyes are closed, and the mouth closed with the lower jaw bound;
  - the body is straightened, with the feet pointing to the door;
  - a candle is lit and placed near the head;
  - mirrors are covered;
  - some orthodox Jews may lay the body on the floor for 20min and pour water outside the door;
  - others may put ashes on the eyes;
- From death until burial, the body is guarded.
- Do not remove any religious objects or threads.

Visiting the home or temple (synagogue)

- Normal social courtesies apply.
- Strict orthodox Jews may prefer not to have home visits on the Sabbath and prefer same-sex doctors and nurses.
- In orthodox synagogues, men and women sit separately, and both men and women cover their heads.

Funeral

- Jews are buried, although some liberal Jews will be cremated.
- The child should be buried within 24h.
- Flowers are not accepted.
- Funerals are simple and unostentatious.
- Gentiles may attend the funeral, but not the internment.
- No mourning is carried out if a baby dies within 30 days of birth.
- The Shiva (7 days of mourning) starts after the burial:
    - three days of private weeping and mourning;
    - then 4 days of shared mourning with friends.
    - prayer of Kaddish said daily;
    - Gentiles are welcome.
- The Sheloshim (30 days) during which the family does not shave or cut their hair. The Kaddish recited daily.
- For the next 10 months, the Kaddish recited weekly by the men.
- Money is given to charity.

Anniversary of death

- On the first anniversary (Yahrzeit), the tombstone is unveiled. Visitors place a small stone on it.
- Yizkor is an annual Jewish holiday when the dead are thought of in a memorial service and candles are lit.

Buddhism

- Buddhists do not worship a God or deities.
- Instead they strive for personal spiritual development to focus on the true meaning of life.
- Their teaching is based on non-violence and compassion for all forms of life.

Symbols and spiritual advisers

- Buddhists may have many religious symbols, but none that are mandatory.
- Spiritual leaders in the community, as well as monks and nuns.

Specific issues

- Buddhists believe in reincarnation.
- Their faith has a strong affinity with death, and they accept death as a process of rebirth, leading to higher levels of enlightenment.
- Their philosophy encompasses the issue of impermanence of life with suffering and, as such, bearing suffering with dignity and equanimity.
- Organ donation and post-mortem are permitted.

Before and after death

- No special requirements.
- As death occurs, local monks and members of the family's local society will say prayers and support the bereaved family.
- The body can be washed.
- It is wrapped in a sheet without emblems.

Visiting the home or temple

- Normal social courtesies apply.

Funeral

- Cremation is the norm, although burial is also permitted.
- There is great variation in the form of the funeral rites, dependent on the Buddhist group.
- There is a calm acceptance of death.

Anniversary of death

- No formal procedure.

Traditional African approaches to a child's death

There is no single 'African approach'. Cultural diversity between southern and northern tribes in Uganda is perhaps greater than between European Caucasians, Australian Aborigines, North American Inuit, and South Asian Indians. Furthermore, in modern Africa, traditional beliefs are often blended with 'Western' religion, so that traditional and Western beliefs regarding health and healing, illness and injury, and death and dying weave inextricably together around the death of children.

Some common beliefs that do span across the different cultures in sub-Saharan Africa, however, have implications for children's palliative care in many diverse African countries and cultures.

Traditional African healing is very much focused on restoring wholeness and peace. 'God' is seen as the ultimate healer and curer and doctor, helped by his divine intermediaries and the good living–dead ancestors, the diviners who can find the cause, the local doctors who can find the cure, and the caring and loving family and community who can make all the above possible. In particular, it tries to restore wholeness and peace between the sick person and:

- God, the ancestors, and the living;
- the family;
- the community and its basic beliefs and values.

Some commonly held beliefs that influence children's palliative care include the following.

- The belief that life is a great gift, and therefore its preservation and prolongation are the central duty of every person, family, and community, which can make it difficult for families to move from a curative to a palliative approach if health workers do not discover and gently challenge it.
- The belief that illness and death (especially in childhood) do not come randomly or independently. Rather, that some enemy (living or dead) must have caused it. This can continue to distract the child and family into searching for external agents and seeking redress, rather than using the limited time left to them in a constructive, peaceful, and supportive way.
- The belief that 'blessings of all sorts come from fulfilling the duty to care for the terminally sick'. This belief sits fairly easily with children's palliative care, as it provides a strong spiritual driver for the family to pull together to do as much as they can to care for the child.
- The belief that a 'good death':
  - comes in old age;
  - is not sudden;
  - allows the patient to make preparations, forgive, and reconcile with all;
  - allows the patient to be able to see their dear ones and bid them farewell.

- Death in childhood is rarely seen as a good death, and the family may need help to focus on all that has been good in a child's life, to feel that life has not been wasted, and to understand that children too have affairs that need to be put in order and farewells that need to be said.
- The belief in the importance of death rituals. Traditional African beliefs put great importance on correct rituals after the death of the child. The particular rituals vary, but there are common themes, particularly around:
  - burying the dead child close to (or within) the family home;
  - not tempting fate by bringing death of very young infants too close to the mother or surviving siblings, in case further childbirth is prevented or surviving children themselves succumb.

In most cases, these rituals seem to serve to complete the circle of life, appease ancestral spirits, and allow the surviving family to move forward unencumbered by unfulfilled obligations from the past.

Ultimately, if a single 'African traditional approach' to healing can be articulated, it is the aim for a sick person to be completely at peace with themselves, to collect together their fears and overcome them, and to be assured that their desires and wishes will be dealt with and that their anxieties and aspirations will be catered for by the ones they love. All these modes of healing are necessary for the children who are dying and their families. Together, they form part of an integrated healing or holistic approach that is culturally appropriate.

Acknowledgement

Special thanks to Dr Narinder Saund and the multifaith group Leicestershire and Dr Justin Amery for the section on traditional African approaches.

Further reading

Murray Parkes, C., Laungani, P., and Young, B. (editors) (2006). *Death and bereavement across cultures*. Routledge, London.

Bereavement

Introduction

It is said that there are only two certainties in life—'death and taxes'. Death is very much part of the normal life cycle of all living creatures. Death generates different levels of grief in people, most often linked to our relationship with the individual and our social cultural upbringing. Up to 100 years ago, in the Western world, death was commonplace and was seen by all age groups. However, in the present day, Western world death is seen much less often and often perceived as a failure of medical technology and skills.

Society and individuals appear to accept the death of the elderly much more easily than the death of a child. The elderly are often seen as having had a good life and achieved many goals. Because our young remain immature and vulnerable for so many years, nature gives us a very powerful parent–child bond. The loss seen with the breaking of the bond generates intense emotion and grief.

As paediatric palliative care professionals dealing with the family, we are looked towards by other health-care professionals and society to help deal with the bereavement and its associated grief. It is important to recognize that it is not our sole responsibility.

- Many cultures have strong religious rituals that are used to support and comfort the family. Many families will look towards their religious community and leaders for support.
- Other families will choose the support within their extended family.
- Finally, the community around a family can be very supportive.

What all these groups lack, because of the small numbers of child deaths, is an understanding of what to expect with the bereavement and how to help with the grief process.

Bereavement theory

Over the last 90 years, the theories around paediatric bereavement have slowly evolved from Freud to the 'stage models', up to our current theories of grief based around 'relearning'. It is helpful to understand the basis of some of these theories. In reality, we use elements from all the theories to help the family.

Stage model

1. Immediately after death: disbelief and denial.
2. Protest phase, with loud crying, motor restlessness, and agitation. Lasting a few weeks or months.
3. Mourning phase where the patient enters a depressive-type phase. Lasting a few months up to the second anniversary of death.
4. Adaptation to the loss.[1–4]

The weakness of this 'medical' model is that it oversimplifies the whole grief process for the parents and family. It compartmentalizes and sets time parameters for the whole process, with a definite end 'when all is well'. In reality, individuals in families grieve at different rates, in different ways, and often flip from one stage to another over time.

Grief work model

- Accepts that grieving takes time and that it is dependent on the individual.
- Grief requires a holistic approach to the individual's needs.
- The individual will need support with personal and emotional issues, as well as help with their interaction with society.
- Gives guidance to caregivers in terms of actively challenging the loss by supporting the 'tasks' of grieving.[5,6]

Relationship with the child model

As with the grief work model, but with additional perspectives:
- the grief process represents an ending of one relationship with the child and the forming of a new relationship with the child;
- the new relationship is long-term;
- the parents continue to remember the child;
- understanding the unique suffering that individuals go through.[7,8]

Bereavement issues for children

The chronically ill child with a life-limiting condition may well experience many personal bereavement issues before their death.
- There is the loss of their normal childhood.
- Loss of the physical ability to do things other children do.
- Loss of the ability to develop normal relationships with school friends and members of the opposite sex.
- Sadness at seeing how hard their parents and families have to struggle to look after them.
- Losses suffered as they see their own health deteriorate, knowing this represents further loss of function of their body, with the threat of death approaching.
- Children with similar medical conditions experience grief, as they see their friends with life-limiting conditions dying around them.

Discussion about death with the child not only helps the child cope with the future, but can also significantly help parents with their bereavement and grief.[9]

Bereavement issues for siblings

Siblings often experience behavioural problems.
- The normal behaviour of siblings is linked to rivalry for parental attention. When their brother or sister has a life-limiting condition, this norm is broken, as the parents concentrate all their attentions on the ill child.
- A large number of siblings develop behavioural problems as a result of bereavement. Research in this group of children is limited. However, the issues that appear to affect their reaction are both general and also developmentally specific.
- Young children tend to be egocentric, so they can sometimes feel that their negative thoughts towards their sibling either caused or exacerbated the sibling's illness.
- Because deaths are rare and children are normally 'protected' by adults, they have limited experience of what a dead person looks like or what their reaction to death should be.
- Children of all ages have vivid imaginations. If no attempt is made to explain, in terms they understand, what is happening to their siblings, then they will start to make up their own ideas from the limited information they hear and based on their limited life experience. As in life, what is imagined is often worse than reality.

Bereavement issues for parents

The way a parent may grieve is dependent on a number of issues.

- The parents' premorbid personality and psychiatric history. Parents with previous anxiety or depression have been shown to be at greater risk of abnormal grief reactions.
- Whether the death was sudden and unexpected, or foreseeable after a prolonged illness. The former group of parents have intense issues with disbelief, denial, and seeking behaviour. The latter group of parents often experience long periods of grief, as they see their child slowly deteriorating.
- Many parents have to combine grief with guilt, particularly when the child may have had a genetic disorder.
- Others find that they need to direct their anger phase at someone—God, their health-care professionals, or spouse.
- Many marriages come under strain and fail, as the couple struggle to remodel their relationship without the child.
- During the illness of a child, many parents lose their normal social circle of friends and family. They replace this with a circle of health-care professionals to whom they become very attached. These same parents feel rejected after the death of a child, as they find the health-care professionals leave to concentrate on the next family. The same happens to social/financial benefits, as they are lost after the child dies, and this can lead to significant financial hardship.
- Religion and ritual can have a great effect on parents' grief reactions (see ➔ Chapter 20). Many benefit greatly from their faiths and the rituals of shared grief with family and friends, particularly around the funeral. Others can find the process distressing if it is imposed on them by the society around them and they have to participate in things with which they do not agree.
- Parents who have a number of children with life-limiting conditions may struggle greatly with grief. They may have already gone through the grief of losing another child. They may have to cope with looking after a sibling knowing that they will have to go through the same grief again in the future.
- In the past, it was felt that, with time, parents would get over the death of their child. Now the thinking is more to do with the parents coming to terms with the death of the child. However, the timescale of this process is uncertain. It was thought in the past to take 1 year, and abnormal grief was diagnosed if it continued for over 2 years. The newer models of grief work and personal experience suggests that rigid time framing is inappropriate. The process of developing a new relationship with the dead child for parents may take years,[10] and abnormal grief should be considered if the parent fails to make progress in the tasks of grieving.

Bereavement issues for society

The death of a child has a profound effect on the community around the child. A great many people are emotionally affected, and it is important to reflect on some of these groups.

Grandparents

The grief felt by grandparents is twofold. Not only do they have to deal with the death of their grandchild, but they also have to deal with the sadness of seeing their own children grieving.

Schools

The death of a child can be a source of great distress to their school friends. For children, this may be their first contact with death. For schoolteachers, there is the difficulty of knowing how to handle the situation.

Managing bereavement

There is a common misconception that child bereavement support needs to come from specialists and counsellors. In reality, this is just not true. Parents obtain most of the support and help through grief from family, friends, and society.[10] Work has shown that normal psychological models of counselling may not be effective.[11,12] However, early support from bereavement support teams can help parents greatly in their grief process.[10] These multidisciplinary teams can help by:

- listening in a non-judgemental way;
- acting as sounding boards for parents, as they try various approaches in the journey through their grief;
- helping parents to maintain a link with the child through memory boxes, etc.;
- helping parents to look at the grief process as a journey of steps, and not something that has to be tackled all in one go;
- supporting parents when things are going badly;
- helping parents through the various emotions of anger, guilt, sadness, and loss;
- helping guide parents as they endeavour to develop new relationships and new ways of working;
- supporting siblings by communication through talking, group work, art therapy, and music therapy—all of these techniques can be used with siblings before, at the time of, and after the death of a child;
- recognizing and embracing the silent suffering seen in grandparents and supporting them through their grief;
- giving advice to schools as to how to approach the issues around death in the school assembly and classroom;
- identifying when grief enters an abnormal phase and initiating specialist medical intervention.

References

1. Bowlby, J. and Parkes, C.M. (1970). Separation and loss within the family. In: Anthony, E.J. and Koupernik, C., editors. *The child in his family*, pp. 197–216. Wiley, New York.
2. Engel, G.L. (1964). Grief and grieving. *Am. J. Nurs.* **64**, 93–8.
3. Osterweis, M., Solomon, F., and Green, M. (1984). *Bereavement: reactions, consequences and care*. National Academy Press, Washington DC.
4. Rosenblatt, P.C., Walsh, R.P., and Jackson, D.A. (1976). *Grief and mourning in cross cultural perspective*. HRAF Press, New Haven.
5. Parkes, C.M. and Weiss, R. (1983). *Recovery from bereavement*. Basic Books, New York.
6. Worden, W. (1991). *Grief counselling and grief therapy: a handbook for the mental health practitioner*, second edition. Springer Publishing Co, New York.
7. Attig, T.W. (1996). *We grieve: relearning the world*. Oxford University Press, New York.
8. Davies, B., Attig, T.W., and Towne, M. (2006). Bereavement. In: Goldman, A., Hain, R., and Liben, S, editors. *Oxford textbook of palliative care for children*, pp. 193–203. Oxford University Press, Oxford.
9. Kreicbergs, U., Valdimarsdottir, U., Henter, J.-I., and Steineck, G. (2004). Talking about death with children who have severe malignant disease. *N. Engl. J. Med.* **351** (12), 1175–86.

10. Kreicbergs, U., Lannen, P., Onelov, E., and Wolfe, J. (2007). Parental grief after losing a child to cancer: impact of professional and social support on long-term outcomes. *J. Clin. Oncol.* **25** (22), 3307–12.

11. Jordan, J.R. and Neimeyer, R.A. (2003). Does grief counselling work? *Death Studies* **27** (9), 765–86.

12. Stroebe, W., Schut, H., and Stroebe, M.S. (2005). Grief work, disclosure and counseling: do they help the bereaved? *Clin. Psychol. Rev.* **25** (4), 395–414.

Chapter 22

Communication skills

Introduction

The medical care of children is characterized by the extent to which it relies on collaboration with family. In effect, the family of a child is expected to behave as colleagues with the paediatric or primary care team. It is expected that they will:

- always be available to the child;
- have the child's best interests at heart;
- be able to work alongside medical and nursing staff.

The goal of communication with patients and families is to ensure the families feel confident and competent in this collegiate relationship (Box 22.1).

Factors that can complicate this include:

- prior understandings and misunderstandings;
- emotional coping mechanisms (e.g. denial);
- discordance between the way information is given and received (e.g. differences in vocabulary between the professional and family);
- difficulty in remembering information.

The aim of communication is twofold:

- to exchange information between the family and professional;
- to minimize the inherent imbalance of power between the professional and lay person in a hospital setting.

Having a structured approach can facilitate those objectives. One approach has five parts:

1. setting the scene;
2. alignment;
3. imparting information;
4. checking;
5. future plans.

Box 22.1 Communication

The goal of good communication is to enable the family of a child or young person to become competent colleagues in his or her medical care through:

- imparting factual information and understanding:
  - to an appropriate level;
  - at an appropriate pace;
  - using appropriate language.
- imparting a sense of participation in the team through:
  - seeking the family's perspective;
  - empathic acknowledgement (implied and overt) of their concerns;
  - soliciting the views of the child and/or family in decision-making.

Setting the scene

- Families find discussions with doctors intimidating and need positive encouragement to volunteer information.
- The aim of setting the scene is to provide a physical and temporal space to facilitate this.
- This usually takes planning. Impromptu communication should be avoided, if possible. It is better to arrange a discussion at a specific time and place.

Physical space

- Privacy. Where possible, a separate room with the door closed. If necessary, at least draw the curtains around the bed.
- A quiet room.
- Comfortable furnishings that allow the professional and family to be on the same physical level.

Temporal space

- Set aside time, ideally by arranging an appointment (and keeping to it).
- Unhurried atmosphere, e.g. by sitting down rather than standing, avoiding talking too fast.
- Minimize interruption, e.g. switch off bleeps and mobile phones.
- Avoid consulting a watch.

Remove barriers

- No desk separating the doctor from the family.
- Eye contact on the same level, emphasizing equality.
- Maintaining eye contact is often interpreted to mean that professionals are not being entirely truthful.

Have the facts straight

- Make sure you feel knowledgeable enough on the subject. If necessary, ask a senior colleague to be present or to facilitate the discussion.
- Do not delegate this important task to inappropriate members of the team (e.g. very junior medical or nursing colleagues).
- Recognize the importance that families give to discussions with doctors.
- Communicate results accurately. If not certain, admit it, rather than risk giving inaccurate information.

Who else should be there?

- Both parents, if possible.
- 'Significant others', e.g. grandparents.
- A member of the nursing staff.
- Consider including the child or young person themselves if you are comfortable.

Alignment

Purpose of alignment

The aim is to understand what things look like from the family's perspective, by establishing what they already know, perceive, and understand. *This means they need to be able to talk first* and to explain:

- what they have already been told;
- their understanding of what they have been told;
- any relevant prior experience and its impact (e.g. the parents of a child newly diagnosed with leukaemia may have had experience of adult cancer that will inform—often erroneously—their understanding of it;
- what vocabulary they use. Insistence on an accurate technical term, in preference to the family's own preferred term (e.g. 'tumour' rather than 'cancer'), risks riding roughshod over important understanding and coping mechanisms, and will compromise the effectiveness of communication.

Tools to assist alignment

- *Open questions* allow the family to set the agenda of the discussion, allowing free rein in interpretation of the question. Open questions can provide rich and varied information, but can jeopardize good communication if they become too unfocused or removed from the point.
- *Closed questions* are used to obtain specific items of information such as 'has anyone in your family had this condition before?'. Overuse of closed questions can restrict discussions and prevent important issues from being addressed. Discussions with no closed questions can be poorly focused and unsatisfactory.
- *Summarizing and checking*—it is important to check that your interpretation of what you are being told is accurate. Summarizing and checking allow this, convey that the physician has listened to what has been said, as well as offer families the opportunity to correct or confirm what has been understood.

Imparting information

A collegiate relationship with families requires them to understand the information you give accurately and to trust that it is truthful. This requires:
- an appropriate level of information;
- information given at an appropriate pace.

Appropriate level of information

Information should:
- be enough to make any necessary decisions in an informed way;
- be enough to allay unnecessary fears;
- be enough to understand the significance of the results of tests that have been done and are immediately planned;
- not overwhelm and obscure what is really important;
- be given using appropriate terminology (avoiding jargon, use family's own terms where possible);
- be relevant. Avoid discussions about increasingly remote possibilities.

The need for information correlates only poorly with perceived educational level. Prior assumptions about a family's intellectual ability risk being patronizing to some and incomprehensibly technical to others.

Appropriate pace

The pace at which information is given should:
- be tailored to the needs of the individual child and family;
- be regulated during the discussion, as new needs become clear;
- be punctuated by summaries, reviews, and a chance to ask questions;
- be supported by written materials (printed or electronic) that can be accessed by families at their own rate.

Checking

Once information has been imparted, ask the family if:
- they have had enough information;
- their concerns have been addressed;
- they have any further questions.

Reassure families that:
- they are not expected to remember everything first time;
- the team is happy to be asked questions again;
- if the consultant is not there, other members of the team, such as nurses on the ward, are able to answer questions.

Be prepared to go over some things again if checking reveals they have not been understood well.

Future plans

Discussions are important to families. Many will feel anxious that the discussion has ended and need to know that there will be future conversations.
- Introduce other members of the team.
- Refer to them during the conversation, so that families recognize that yours is not the only expert voice.
- Ditto the primary care team if the child is to be discharged home.
- Make a further appointment to meet the family at a certain date or time.
- Be honest if there is the possibility that you will be late.
- Ensure that your plans for meeting again are acceptable to the family, particularly if the child is to be discharged.

Summary of communication skills
- Discussion of bad news begins with a process of finding out how the situation is seen by the patient and family.
- This is followed by a period when the doctor gives information at a pace, level, and amount that the family can assimilate accurately and easily.
- Check for understanding at intervals throughout the discussion and on completion.
- Repeat information, if necessary.
- Make future plans, including arrangements for any follow-up meeting.

Chapter 23

Communication amongst professionals

Introduction

Communication skills amongst professionals all centre on the basic ideology of teamworking. Teamworking has repeatedly been shown in both business and health to be effective. The WHO affirms that primary health should involve all related sectors working together, including education and social services, in addition to health care, and that efforts should be made to coordinate these sectors.[1]

General points

- Teamworking can only work effectively when the child and family are seen as central to the 'team', with all the professionals acting as spokes to the central hub of family (Fig. 23.1).
- On average, a disabled child has contact with ten different professionals and attends 20 clinic visits a year.[2]
- All the children who require palliative care will have different requirements, but, in common, they need everyone to work together and be clear on their roles and responsibilities, to ensure that the child's and family's needs are met in a supportive and timely manner.

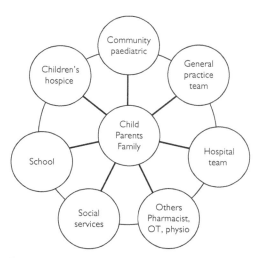

Fig. 23.1 Professional involvement in the care of a child.

Definitions

Teamworking can be defined as 'a group of individuals who share goals and work together to deliver services for which they are mutually accountable'.

A variety of terms are used relating to the structure and philosophy of the teams; these include multidisciplinary, interdisciplinary, and transdisciplinary. These terms are not interchangeable but instead represent different forms of communication within teams.

Multidisciplinary teamworking

In multidisciplinary teamworking, professionals collaborate and cooperate, but within their own set roles.
- Various professional groups meet together.
- Those with varying knowledge and skill bases meet together within a single agency.
- Different agencies meet together.

Interdisciplinary teamworking

In interdisciplinary teamworking, there is adaptation of roles and responsibilities, etc. to adjust to those of others in the team. This allows for integration of theoretical models and techniques.
- Professionals adapt their identified roles to interact with, and take account of, others in the group.
- There are adjustments to knowledge and skill bases.
- This results in various agency responsibilities.

Transdisciplinary teamworking

In transdisciplinary teamworking, there is a reformation of roles, knowledge, and skills to create family-centred cohesive services, with only one assessment.

Team theory

A number of authors have written about how a team forms (Table 23.1). The pattern that emerges from all these models is that a team develops over time, as individuals learn about each other's skill and knowledge. Roles are defined, and responsibility is delegated. Conflict appears to be a natural event in the evolution of the team.

Handy[3] identified the factors required to develop a successful team (Table 23.2).

Table 23.1 Models for the development of teams

Lowe[4]	Roelofsen et al.[5]	Handy[3]
Becoming acquainted	Process-oriented	Forming
Trial and error	Result-oriented	Storming
Collective indecision	Problem-oriented	Norming
Crisis	Interdisciplinary team	Performing
Resolution		

Table 23.2 Factors for a successful team

The givens	
The group	Size, member characteristics, individual objectives, and stage of development
The task	Nature of the task; criteria of effectiveness, salience of the task, and clarity of the task
The environment	Norms and expectations, the leader position, intergroup relations, and the physical location
Intervening factors	Leadership style
	Process and procedure
	Motivation
Outcomes	Productivity
	Member satisfaction

Challenges of teamworking

There are considerable challenges involved in teamworking, particularly when one also looks at joint working at broader levels, including strategic planning and service commissioning.

Organizational challenges
- Many organizations have their own way of working, hierarchy, pay, funding, geography, and training.
- Organizations have different ideologies, cultures, and attitudes.
- Organizational rigidity.
- Different levels of commitment.
- Time factors.
- Differing perceptions of the value of liaison.
- Attitude to leadership.
- Lack of training in teamworking or leadership skills.
- Power struggles over control and funding.
- Issues over justice of allocation of limited resources.
- Issues about individuals and the organizational value of their status or importance.
- Conflict can occur when either party does not complete their expected role and responsibilities, or blocks completion of goals set by others.
- Lack of understanding of the skills and roles of each other's profession.

Communication problems
- Communication problems within each agency and also between them.
- Lack of understanding of the need to communicate with particular groups, in particular, teachers, schools, and education.
- Use of language by professionals, particularly use of complex medical terms.
- Different interpretation of common language by different professionals, e.g. 'patient-centred', 'collaboration', or 'advocacy'.
- The complexity and rarity of the types of medical conditions means that knowledge of the conditions is restricted to a limited number of tertiary care specialist experts.

'Too many cooks'

Large numbers of professionals can be involved in looking after an individual child and family, particularly within the first year of diagnosis. The repeated contact by all these workers puts a major strain on the family and child, in terms of coordination, communication, understanding roles, developing relationships, and assessing which services are available. Parents will often complain that they feel swamped and suffocated by the number of people from the 'caring professions' they have to meet. The number of people involved can lead to inertia and confusion over care and responsibilities.

Successful teamworking

Although there are many challenges, with some effort, we can still establish good effective teamworking.[4–6]

- Planning ahead.
- Appropriate design and membership of the team.
- Allocation of time and funds.
- Appropriate location, facilities, and resources for the team.
- Good leadership based on skill, rather than perceived status.
- Ability to change leadership, as the needs of the child and family change.
- Leader able to coordinate individuals and organizations.
- Members to understand their own role and that of other members of the group.
- Respect for each other's knowledge and experience.
- Focused allocation of responsibilities and workload.
- Flexibility and compromise.
- Aim to set clear goals that are appropriate, specific, and measurable.
- Information to be disseminated in a clear understandable form to all members of the team, child, and family.

Key worker

The identification of an appropriate person to act as key worker and as a coordinator is one suggestion to achieve effective teamwork to meet the palliative care needs of a child and family.

Some specific roles of a key worker have been identified, which include:

- information provision;
- identifying and addressing the child's and family's needs;
- coordinating timely services;
- emotional support;
- acting in the role of advocate.

As with all services, the balance of these roles is dependent on the individual needs of the family and child. The key worker, in effect, takes on the role of 'team leader' for that child and family.

References

1. World Health Organization (1978). *Declaration of Alma-Ata.* World Health Organization, Geneva.
2. Department of Health (2004). *National services framework for children, young people and maternity services. Disabled children and young people and those with complex health needs.* Department of Health, London. Available at: ℘ https://www.gov.uk/government/uploads/system/uploads/attachment_data/file/199955/National_Service_Framework_for_Children_Young_People_and_Maternity_Services_-_Disabled_Children_and_Young_People_and_those_with_Complex_Health_Needs.pdf.
3. Handy, C. (1993). On the workings of groups. In: Handy, C. *Understanding organizations,* fourth edition, pp. 150–79. Penguin, London.
4. Lowe, J. and Herranen, M. (1978). Conflict in teamworking. *Soc. Work Health Care* 3 (3), 323–30.
5. Roelofsen, E.E., The, B.A., Beckerman, H., Lankhorst, G.J., and Bouter, L.M. (2002). Development and implementation of the Rehabilitation Activities Profile for children: impact on the rehabilitation team. *Clin. Rehabil.* 16 (4), 441–53.

6. Watson, D., Townsley, R., Abbott, D., and Latham, P. (2002). *Working together? Multi-agency working in services to disabled children with complex health care needs and their families. A literature review.* Handsel Trust Publications, Birmingham.
7. Watson, D., Townsley, R., and Abbot, D. (2002). Exploring multi-agency working in services to disabled children with complex healthcare needs and their families. *J. Clin. Nurs.* **11**, 365–75.
8. Pardess, E., Finzi, R., and Sever, J. (1993). Evaluating the best interests of the child—a model of multidisciplinary teamwork. *Med. Law* **12** (3–5), 205–11.

Coping skills

Introduction

Working within health care induces different levels of stress in professionals. When dealing with life-limited children, these stresses can be immense
and, if not managed correctly, can lead to burnout.

Issues

Some of the issues that health-care professionals may face involve the
following:[1]

- their own feelings around advancing disease and death, and the impact
  this work has on the practitioners and their family;
- their ability to recognize, reflect on, and deal with conflicts of belief and
  values within the team;
- their ability to work to resolve conflicts when they arise;
- their ability to recognize and manage their own personality, reactions,
  and emotions constructively in relation to self, patients, and colleagues;
- their ability to manage anger;
- their ability to give and receive criticism constructively;
- their ability to manage uncertainty and the unexpected, make difficult
  decisions, and multitask;
- their ability to recognize stress, mental ill health, and burnout in self and
  other professionals;
- their ability to ask for help and hand over to others appropriately, and
  their ability to use a range of methods to receive support from, and give
  support to, colleagues;
- their ability to recognize and deal competently with potential sources of
  difficulty, including:
  - over-involvement;
  - personal identification;
  - negative feelings and personality clashes;
  - demands that cannot be met.
- effective time management and the ability to prioritize effectively.

Management

The key to successful management of these issues is awareness of the problems and pre-planning of the solutions.

- It is important to have communication and support mechanisms built into any organization.
- The health-care professional should know their capabilities through the process of reflective practice and discussion with colleagues.
- There should be an openness to consult other professionals to seek advice.
- Realistic goals and expectations need to be set when planning care for a child.
- The doctor, team, and family need to understand that, by definition of a terminal illness, treatments may fail and need to be adjusted continually.
- Parental reactions to the death of a child are very varied. Occasionally, the parents need to vent these emotions, and this is sometimes directed towards a health-care professional. This should not be seen as a personal attack, but more of a reflection of the frustration the parent is feeling at the time. It can be helpful to ask the question 'how can we help these parents', rather than labelling them as being awkward.
- Teamworking can be difficult, and team dynamics change over time. It is helpful to understand the theory of team building to understand that conflict can be a positive influence in building a team.
- Organizational culture should develop where criticism is seen as a positive opportunity to address issues and raise standards, and not negatively to put people down. This can only happen if feedback is given in a constructive, respectful, and honest way.
- The professional should consider having a mentoring system to allow for an opportunity to discuss issues. If a formal system is not available, then having an equal colleague to whom one can talk informally can be helpful.
- All organizations should have a system of debrief after the death of a child. This allows the team to share an outlet of emotions in a controlled environment. This debrief needs to be led by an experienced member of the team.
- It is important to have built into the structure of any team an independent occupational health facility and also anonymous direct access to counselling.
- To be emotionally affected by the death of a child and even cry a few tears is normal; conversely, just because someone does not cry does not mean they have not been moved by the experience. However, to lose emotional control completely is damaging to the individual, their colleagues, and the family. Sadly, once we finish with one child, there is always a list of others waiting for our professional input.
- Paediatric palliative care cannot be done in a hurry. The average palliative care assessment takes 1–2h. For the parents, the fact that their child is dying makes them a priority over everything and everyone else when things are going wrong. Any attempt to hurry the consultation or to 'fob them off' is perceived very badly and is a particularly common complaint.

- Once a health-care professional reaches a stage of feeling overloaded, the system should allow them to step back from front line work to recharge.
- Paediatric palliative care is not easy and is not something every professional can do. When it becomes apparent that an individual cannot face the emotional impact of this type of work, they should be allowed to leave without any sense of failure.

Reference

1. Bild, R. and Gómez, I. (2014). *An unwanted journey: creative accompaniment in paediatric palliative care*. Plamienok Books.

Chapter 25

Education and training

Background

- PPM was recognized in the UK as a subspecialty of paediatrics in 2009.
- Unusually amongst paediatric subspecialties, PPM is defined by the needs of individual patients, rather than by their diagnosis or diseased organ system (which may indeed not be known).
- The intention of developing a curriculum is to set a standard for improvement.
- Children's hospices require palliative care skills for children rooted both in primary care and in paediatrics. This interface with primary care is an important and unique part of PPM training.

Levels of training

In PPM, four levels of competence are currently described.

- *Level 1* (expected from all newly qualified doctors). *Understand basic principles of palliative care.*
- *Level 2* (expected of all those completing their core paediatric training). *Apply basic principles to the care of children, and recognize reversible causes.*
- *Level 3* (consultant paediatrician with special interest in palliative medicine). *Be able to manage most common symptoms, but recognize the need to consult a tertiary specialist when appropriate. Often achieved through postgraduate Diploma/MSc and/or SPIN training.*
- *Level 4* (tertiary specialist in PPM). *Have completed a 2-year national grid training programme in PPM.*

Paediatric palliative medicine curriculums

By definition, a curriculum comprises:
- a set of competencies in the subject;
- a set of tools to evaluate them.

Competencies

Formal and systematic training is essential if gaps in knowledge, skills, and attitude are to be recognized and rectified by those working, or hoping to work, in children's palliative care. Thorough training in medical care of sick children (e.g. completion of core paediatric Specialist Registrar training) is a prerequisite but is not sufficient in itself. Palliative medicine is recognized by the UK RCPCH as a subspecialty within paediatrics.

Royal College of Paediatrics and Child Health

The RCPCH sets out competencies required from paediatricians who have completed specialist training in palliative medicine that will allow them a certificate of specialist training in paediatrics/palliative medicine:
- specifies competencies unique to palliative medicine (i.e. different from general paediatric competencies);
- based on the Association for Paediatric Palliative Medicine (APPM) curriculum (see ➲ Association for Paediatric Palliative Medicine below);
- forms basis for subspecialty (GRID) training in PPM and also for special interest (SPIN) training;
- available to trainees from the RCPCH website (℗ www.rcpch.ac.uk).

RCPCH-approved training is coordinated by a Specialist Advisory Committee in PPM and delivered through a series of GRID and SPIN posts across the UK, to which paediatric trainees are appointed centrally through a competitive interview process.

Association for Paediatric Palliative Medicine

The APPM has defined competencies in PPM that should be expected from all doctors.
- Comprehensive set of PPM competencies, including those in common with other specialties.
- Not restricted to PPM specialists but includes competencies expected of all doctors.
- Available, without cost, from the APPM website (℗ http://appm.org.uk/14.html).
- Defines four levels of specialization:
  - all qualifying doctors;
  - all paediatricians;
  - paediatricians or GPs with an interest in PPM;
  - specialists in PPM.

Other national curriculums
- PPM Diploma/MSc in Palliative Medicine (Cardiff University)
(℞ http://courses.cardiff.ac.uk/postgraduate/course/detail/p233.html).
- Education in Palliative and End-of-life Care (EPEC, North America)
(℞ http://www.epec.net).
- Royal College of Physicians (UK). Adult physicians training in palliative medicine are expected to have some knowledge of the paediatric specialty.

Evaluation tools
All subspecialty paediatric training in the UK, including PPM, is assessed formatively, using the same series of evaluation tools. They are constantly being reviewed and are listed on ℞ http://www.rcpch.ac.uk/training-examinations-professional-development/assessment-and-examinations/assessment/assessment.

Additional evaluation tools that are specific to the subspecialty of palliative medicine include:
- communication skills assessment by observation and video;
- structured portfolio of case reports;
- relevant clinical audits;
- structured examination questions.

Summary of education and training
- Competencies in PPM overlap with those in other paediatric specialties, as well as with adult palliative medicine and primary care.
- All doctors should know something about PPM.
- Four levels of training have been defined that encompass expertise from graduating physicians to trained subspecialists.
- There is a small, but growing, number of curriculums in PPM, each of which consists of a set of competencies and a set of evaluation tools.

Further reading

Association for Paediatric Palliative Medicine Education Subgroup, Paediatric Palliative Medicine College Specialty Advisory Committee (Royal College of Paediatrics and Child Health) (2015). *Curriculum in paediatric palliative medicine*, second edition. Together for Short Lives, Bristol. Available at: ℞ http://appm.org.uk/14.html.

Ferguson, L., Fowler-Kerry, S., and Hain, R.D.W. (2012). Education. In: Goldman, A., Hain, R., and Liben, S., editors. *Oxford textbook of palliative care for children*, second edition, pp. 420–9. Oxford University Press, Oxford (also available on-line).

Friedrichsdorf, S.J., Wolfe, J., Remke, S., Hauser, J., Foster, L., and Emanuel, L., editors. (2015). *The education in palliative and end-of-life care for pediatrics curriculum*. EPEC®-Pediatrics.

Hain, R.D.W. (2016). Palliative care. In: Lissauer, T. and Carroll, W., editors. *The science of paediatrics: MRCPCH mastercourse*. Elsevier Health Sciences, London.

Formulary

Adrenaline (topical)

Uses
Small external bleeds.

Dose and routes
Soak gauze in 1:1000 (1mg/mL) solution, and apply directly to bleeding point.

Alfentanil

Uses
- Short-acting, synthetic, lipophilic, opioid analgesic derivative of fentanyl.
- Used as analgesic, especially intraoperatively and for patients in intensive care and on assisted ventilation (adjunct to anaesthesia).
- Alternative opioid if intolerant to other strong opioids; useful in renal failure if neurotoxic on morphine, or stages 4–5 severe renal failure.
- Useful for breakthrough pain and procedure-related pain.

Dose and routes
- Analgesic, especially intraoperatively and for patients in intensive care and on assisted ventilation (adjunct to anaesthesia). SEEK SPECIALIST ADVICE.
- By iv/sc bolus (*these doses assume* assisted ventilation is available):
  - *neonate*: 5–20 micrograms/kg initial dose, supplemental doses up to 10 micrograms/kg;
  - *1 month to 18 years*: 10–20 micrograms/kg initial dose, up to 10 micrograms/kg supplemental doses.
- By continuous iv or sc infusion (*these doses assume* assisted ventilation is available):
  - *neonate*: 10–50 micrograms/kg over 10min, then 30–60 micrograms/kg/h;
  - *1 month to 18 years*: 50–100 micrograms/kg loading dose over 10min, then 30–60 micrograms/kg/h as a continuous infusion.
- Alternative opioid if intolerant to other strong opioids; useful in renal failure if neurotoxic on morphine, or stages 4–5 severe renal failure. SEEK SPECIALIST ADVICE.
- Doses should be based on opioid equivalence, with the following suggested as safe and practical conversion ratios.
- po morphine to continuous subcutaneous infusion (CSCI) alfentanil: 1/30th of the 24h total po morphine dose, e.g. 60mg/24h po morphine = 2mg/24h CSCI alfentanil.
- CSCI/iv morphine to CSCI alfentanil: 1/15th of the 24h total CSCI/iv morphine dose, e.g. 30mg/24h CSCI/iv morphine = 2mg/24h CSCI alfentanil.
- CSCI diamorphine to CSCI alfentanil: 1/10th of the 24h total diamorphine dose, e.g. 30mg/24h diamorphine = 3mg/24h CSCI alfentanil.

- If conversion is due to toxicity of the previous opioid, lower doses of alfentanil may be needed to provide adequate analgesia.
- *Opioid-naïve adults*: CSCI 500 micrograms to 1mg over 24h.

Breakthrough pain
SEEK SPECIALIST ADVICE.
- sc/sublingual/buccal.
- Suggest 1/6th to 1/10th of the total CSCI dose. However, there is a poor relationship between the effective prn dose and the regular background dose. Alfentanil has a short duration of action (~30min), and, even with an optimally titrated prn dose, frequent dosing (even every 1–2h) may be required. Dose and frequency of administration should be regularly reviewed.

Procedure-related pain
SEEK SPECIALIST ADVICE.
- sc/sublingual/buccal.
- *Adults*: 250–500 micrograms, single dose.
- *Child*: 5 micrograms/kg, single dose.

Give dose 5min before an event likely to cause pain; repeat, if needed.

Notes
- Alfentanil injection is licensed for use in children as an analgesic supplement for use before and during anaesthesia. Use for pain relief in palliative care is unlicensed. Buccal, sublingual, or intranasal administration of alfentanil for incident/breakthrough pain is an unlicensed indication and route of administration. The injection solution may be used for buccal, sublingual, or intranasal administration (unlicensed).
- There is limited information/evidence for analgesic doses in palliative care, especially in children. Doses are largely extrapolated from suggested equianalgesic doses with other opioids.
- Potency: 10–20 times stronger than parenteral morphine, ~25% of the potency of fentanyl.
- Very useful in patients with severe renal failure (no dose reduction is needed). May need to reduce the dose in severe hepatic impairment.
- In order to avoid excessive dosage in obese children, the dose may need to be calculated on the basis of ideal weight for height, rather than actual weight.
- Pharmacokinetics: half-life is prolonged in neonates, so can accumulate in prolonged use. Clearance may be increased from 1 month to 12 years of age, so higher infusion doses may be needed.
- Contraindication: not to be administered concurrently with monoamine oxidase inhibitors (MAOIs) or within 2 weeks of their discontinuation.
- Interaction: alfentanil levels are increased by inhibitors of cytochrome P450.

- Adverse effects include respiratory depression, hypotension, hypothermia, muscle rigidity (which can be managed with neuromuscular-blocking drugs).
- For sc or iv infusion, alfentanil is compatible with 0.9% sodium chloride (NaCl) or 5% glucose as a diluent. For CSCI alfentanil, appears compatible with most drugs used in a syringe driver. Like diamorphine, high doses of alfentanil may be dissolved in small volumes of diluent, which is very useful for sc administration.
- Available as: injection (500 micrograms/mL in 2mL and 10mL ampoules); intensive care injection (5mg/mL in 1mL ampoules which must be diluted before use). Nasal spray with attachment for buccal/sublingual use (5mg/5mL bottle available as special order from Torbay Hospital: each 'spray' delivers 0.14mL = 140 micrograms alfentanil).

Amitriptyline

Uses
- Neuropathic pain.

Dose and routes
By mouth
- *Child 2–12 years*: initial dose of 200 micrograms/kg (maximum 10mg), given od at night. Dose may be increased gradually, if necessary, to a suggested maximum of 1mg/kg/dose twice daily (bd) (under specialist supervision).
- *Child 12–18 years*: initial dose of 10mg at night, increased gradually, if necessary, every 3–5 days to a suggested initial maximum of 75mg/day. Higher doses up to 150mg/day in divided doses may be used under specialist advice.

Notes
- Not licensed for use in children with neuropathic pain.
- Analgesic effect unlikely to be evident for several days. Potential improved sleep and appetite which are likely to precede analgesic effect.
- Drug interactions: not to be administered concurrently with MAOIs or within 2 weeks of their discontinuation. Caution with concurrent use of drugs which inhibit or induce CYP2D6 enzymes.
- Main side effects limiting use in children include constipation, dry mouth, and drowsiness.
- Liquid may be administered via an enteral feeding tube.
- Available as: tablets (10mg, 25mg, 50mg) and oral solution (25mg/5mL, 50mg/5mL).

Aprepitant

Uses
- Prevention and treatment of nausea and vomiting associated with emetogenic cancer chemotherapy.

Dose and routes
For oral administration
- *Child <10 years*: 3mg/kg (max 125mg) as a single dose on Day 1 (1h before chemotherapy), followed by 2mg/kg (max 80mg) as a single dose on Day 2 and Day 3.
- *Child >10 years*: 125mg as a single dose on Day 1 (1h before chemotherapy), followed by 80mg as a single dose on Day 2 and Day 3.

Aprepitant is used in combination with a corticosteroid (usually dexamethasone) and a $5HT_3$ antagonist such as ondansetron.

Notes
- Aprepitant is licensed for the prevention of acute and delayed nausea and vomiting associated with highly or moderately emetogenic cancer chemotherapy in adults.
- Aprepitant is not licensed for use in children and adolescents less than 18 years of age (although a number of clinical trials are currently ongoing). Limited evidence for use in those less than 10 years of age.
- Aprepitant is a selective high-affinity antagonist at NK_1 receptors.
- Aprepitant is a substrate, a moderate inhibitor, and inducer of the CYP3A4 isoenzyme system. It is also an inducer of CYP2C9 and therefore has the potential to interact with any other drugs that are also metabolized by these enzyme systems, including rifampicin, carbamazepine, phenobarbital, itraconazole, clarithromycin, warfarin, and dexamethasone. Please note this list is not exhaustive—seek advice.
- Common side effects include hiccups, dyspepsia, diarrhoea, constipation, anorexia, asthenia, headache, and dizziness.
- Available as: capsules 80mg and 125mg. A formulation for extemporaneous preparation of an oral suspension is available.

Arachis oil enema

Uses
- Faecal softener.
- Faecal impaction.

Dose and routes
By rectal administration
- *Child 3–7 years*: 45–65mL as required (~1/3 to 1/2 enema).
- *Child 7–12 years*: 65–100mL as required (~1/2 to 3/4 enema).
- *Child 12 years and over*: 100–130mL as required (~3/4 to 1 enema).

Notes
- Caution: as arachis oil is derived from peanuts, do not use in children with a known allergy to peanuts.
- Generally used as a retention enema to soften impacted faeces. May be instilled and left overnight to soften the stool.
- Warm the enema before use by placing in warm water.
- Administration may cause local irritation.
- Licensed for use in children from 3 years of age.
- Available as: enema, arachis (peanut) oil in 130mL single-dose disposable packs.

Aspirin

Uses
- Mild to moderate pain.
- Pyrexia.

Dose and routes
By mouth
- *>16 years of age*: initial dose of 300mg every 4–6h when necessary. Dose may be increased, if necessary, to a maximum of 900mg every 4–6h (maximum 4g/day).

Notes
- Contraindicated in children due to risk of Reye's syndrome.
- Use with caution in asthma, previous peptic ulceration, severe hepatic or renal impairment.
- May be used in low dose under specialist advice for children with some cardiac conditions.
- Available as: tablets (75mg, 300mg), dispersible tablets (75mg, 300mg), and suppositories (150mg available from special-order manufacturers or specialist importing companies).

Baclofen

Uses
- Chronic severe spasticity of voluntary muscle.
- Considered as third-line neuropathic agent.

Dose and routes
By mouth
- *Initial dose for child under 18 years*: 300 micrograms/kg/day in four divided doses (maximum single dose 2.5mg), increased gradually at weekly intervals to a usual maintenance dose of 0.75–2mg/kg/day in divided doses, with the following maximum daily doses:
  - *child up to 8 years*: maximum total daily dose 40mg/day;
  - *child 8–18 years*: maximum total daily dose 60mg/day.

Notes
- Review treatment if no benefit within 6 weeks of achieving maximum dose.
- There are very limited clinical data on the use of baclofen in children under the age of 1 year. Use in this patient population should be based on the physician's consideration of individual benefit and risk of therapy.
- Monitor and review reduction in muscle tone and potential adverse effects on swallow and airway protection.
- Avoid abrupt withdrawal.
- Intrathecal use by specialist only.
- Risk of toxicity in renal impairment; use smaller oral doses and increase dosage interval, if necessary.
- Contraindicated if there is a history of active peptic ulceration.
- Administration with or after food may minimize gastric irritation.
- May be administered via enteral feeding tubes. Use a liquid formulation for small doses; dilute prior to use to reduce viscosity. Consider dispersing tablets in water for higher doses, owing to the sorbitol content of the liquid formulation.
- Available as: tablets (10mg) and oral solution (5mg/5mL).

Bethanechol

Uses
- Opioid-induced urinary retention.

Dose and routes
By mouth
- *Child over 1 year*: 0.6mg/kg/day in three or four divided doses. Maximum single dose 10mg.
- *Adult dose*: 10–25mg per dose 3–4 times a day. Occasionally, it may be felt necessary to initiate therapy with a 50mg dose.

Subcutaneous
- *Child over 1 year*: 0.12–2mg/kg/day in three or four divided doses. Maximum single dose 2.5mg.
- *Adult dose*: 2.5–5mg per dose 3–4 times a day.

Notes
- The safety and efficacy of bethanechol in children have not been established (bethanechol is not licensed for use in children).
- Preferably taken before food to reduce the potential for nausea and vomiting.
- Contraindicated in hyperthyroidism, peptic ulcer, asthma, cardiac disease, and epilepsy.
- Tablets may be crushed and dispersed in water for administration via an enteral feeding tube; a formulation for extemporaneous oral suspension is available.
- Available as: tablets (10mg and 25mg), injection for sc injection only (5mg/mL—not licensed in the UK but may be possible to import via a specialist importation company).

Bisacodyl

Uses
- Constipation.

Dose and routes
By mouth
- *Child 4–18 years*: 5–20mg od; adjust according to response.

By rectum (suppository)
- *Child 2–18 years*: 5–10mg od; adjust according to response.

Notes
- Tablets act in 10–12h. Suppositories act in 20–60min; suppositories must be in direct contact with the mucosal wall.
- Stimulant laxative.
- Prolonged or excessive use can cause electrolyte disturbance.
- Available as: tablets (5mg) and suppositories (5mg, 10mg).

Buprenorphine

Uses
- Moderate to severe pain.

Dose and routes
By sublingual route (starting doses)
- *Child body weight 16–25kg*: 100 micrograms every 6–8h.
- *Child body weight 25–37.5kg*: 100–200 micrograms every 6–8h.
- *Child body weight 37.5–50kg*: 200–300 micrograms every 6–8h.
- *Child body weight over 50kg*: 200–400 micrograms every 6–8h.

By transdermal patch
- By titration or as indicated by existing opioid needs.

Buprenorphine patches are *approximately* equivalent to the following 24h doses of po morphine.

Morphine salt 12mg daily ≡	BuTrans® '5' patch	7-day patches
Morphine salt 24mg daily ≡	BuTrans® '10' patch	7-day patches
Morphine salt 48mg daily ≡	BuTrans® '20' patch	7-day patces
Morphine salt 84mg daily ≡	Transtec® '35' patch	4-day patches
Morphine salt 126mg daily ≡	Transtec® '52.5' patch	4-day patches
Morphine salt 168mg daily ≡	Transtec® '70' patch	4-day patches

Notes
- Sublingual tablets not licensed for use in children <6 years old.
- Patches not licensed for use in children.
- Has both opioid agonist and antagonist properties, and may precipitate withdrawal symptoms, including pain, in children dependent on high doses of other opioids.
- Sublingual duration of action 6–8h.
- Caution with hepatic impairment and potential interaction with many drugs, including antiretrovirals.
- Available as tablets (200 micrograms, 400 micrograms) for sublingual administration. Tablets may be halved.
- Available as three types of patches:
  - BuTrans®—applied every 7 days. Available as 5 (5 micrograms/h for 7 days),10 (10 micrograms/h for 7 days), and 20 (20 micrograms/h for 7 days);
  - Transtec®—applied every 96h. Available as 35 (35 micrograms/h for 96h), 52.5 (52.5 micrograms/h for 96h), and 70 (70 micrograms/h for 96h).
  - Hapoctasin®—available as 35, 52.5 and 70 micrograms/h for 72 hours.
- For patches, systemic analgesic concentrations are generally reached within 12–24h, but levels continue to rise for 32–54h. If converting from:
  - 4-hourly po morphine—give regular doses for the first 12h after applying the patch;
  - 12-hourly slow-release morphine—apply the patch, and give the final slow-release dose at the same time;
  - 24-hourly slow-release morphine—apply the patch 12h after the final slow-release dose;
  - CSCI—continue the syringe driver for about 12h after applying the patch.
- Effects only partially reversed by naloxone.
- Rate of absorption from patches is affected by temperature, so caution with pyrexia or increased external temperature such as hot baths—possibility of accidental overdose, with respiratory depression.
- Patches are finding a use as an easily administered option for low-dose background opioid analgesia in a stable situation, for example in severe neurological impairment.
- Schedule 3 controlled drug (CD).

Carbamazepine

Uses
- Neuropathic pain.
- Some movement disorders.
- Anticonvulsant.

Dose and routes

By mouth

- *Child 1 month to 12 years*: initial dose of 5mg/kg at night or 2.5mg/kg bd, increased, as necessary, by 2.5–5mg/kg every 3–7 days, usual maintenance dose; 5mg/kg 2–3 times daily. Doses up to 20mg/kg/day in divided doses have been used.
- *Child 12–18 years*: initial dose of 100–200mg 1–2 times daily; increased slowly to usual maintenance of 200–400mg 2–3 times daily. Maximum 1.8g/day in divided doses.

By rectum

- *Child 1 month to 18 years*: use ~25% more than the oral dose (maximum single dose 250mg) up to four times daily (qds).

Notes

- Not licensed for use in children with neuropathic pain.
- Can cause serious blood, hepatic, and skin disorders. Parents should be taught how to recognize signs of these conditions, particularly leucopenia.
- Numerous interactions with other drugs, including chemotherapy drugs.
- Different preparations may vary in bioavailability, so avoid changing formulations or brands.
- Suppositories of 125mg are approximately equivalent to 100mg tablets.
- Oral liquid has been administered pr—should be retained for at least 2h, if possible, but may have a laxative effect.
- For administration via an enteral feeding tube, use the liquid preparation. Dilute with an equal volume of water immediately prior to administration. If giving doses higher than 400mg/day, divide into four equal doses.
- Available as: tablets (100mg, 200mg, 400mg), chew tablets (100mg, 200mg), liquid (100mg/5mL), suppositories (125mg, 250mg), and modified-release tablets (200mg, 400mg).

Celecoxib

Uses

- Pain, inflammatory pain, bone pain, stiffness. Not used first-line.
- Dose based on management of juvenile rheumatoid arthritis.

Dose and routes

By mouth

- *Child over 2 years*:
  - weight 10–25kg: 50mg bd or 100mg daily;
  - weight >25kg: 100mg bd.

Notes

- Celecoxib is a cyclo-oxygenase-2 (COX-2) selective inhibitor.
- Not licensed in the UK for use in children.
- All NSAID use (including COX-2 selective inhibitors) can, to varying degrees, be associated with a small increased risk of thrombotic events (e.g. myocardial infarction and stroke), independent of baseline cardiovascular risk factors or duration of NSAID use; however, the greatest risk may be in those receiving high doses long-term. COX-2 inhibitors are associated with an increased risk of thrombotic effects.
- All NSAIDs are associated with serious gastrointestinal toxicity. COX-2 inhibitors are associated with a *lower risk* of serious upper gastrointestinal side effects than non-selective NSAIDs.
- Use with caution in patients with renal impairment, and avoid in severe renal impairment.
- Use with caution in hepatic impairment.
- Celecoxib interacts with a great many commonly used drugs; check the *British National Formulary* (*BNF*) (current version online).
- Capsules may be opened, and contents mixed with soft food immediately before administration. For a 50mg dose, approximately halve the 100mg capsule contents to give the best estimate of a 50mg dose.
- Available as: capsules 100mg, 200mg.

Chloral hydrate

Uses

- Insomnia.
- Agitation.

Dose and routes

By mouth or rectum

- *Neonate*: initial dose of 30mg/kg as a single dose at night. May be increased to 45mg/kg at night or when required.
- *Child 1 month to 12 years*: initial dose of 30mg/kg as a single dose at night. May be increased to 50mg/kg at night or when required. Maximum single dose 1g.
- *Child 12–18 years*: initial dose of 500mg as a single dose at night or when required. Dose may be increased, if necessary, to 1–2g. Maximum single dose 2g.

Notes

- Not licensed in agitation or in infants <2 years for insomnia.
- Oral use: mix with plenty of juice, water, or milk to reduce gastric irritation and disguise the unpleasant taste.
- For rectal administration, use oral solution or suppositories (available from 'specials' manufacturers).
- Accumulates on prolonged use and should be avoided in severe renal or hepatic impairment.

- Available as: tablets (chloral betaine 707mg = choral hydrate 414mg—Welldorm®), oral solution (143.3mg/5mL—Welldorm®; 200mg/5mL, 500mg/5mL, both of which are available from 'specials' manufacturers or specialist importing companies), and suppositories (available as various strengths—25mg, 50mg, 60mg, 100mg, 200mg, 500mg, from 'specials' manufacturers).

Chlorpromazine

Uses
- Hiccups.
- Nausea and vomiting of terminal illness (where other drugs are unsuitable).

Dose and routes
Hiccups

By mouth
- *Child 1–6 years*: 500 micrograms/kg every 4–6h, adjusted according to response (maximum 40mg daily).
- *Child 6–12 years*: 10mg three times daily (tds), adjusted according to response (maximum 75mg daily).
- *Child 12–18 years*: 25mg tds (or 75mg at night), adjusted according to response; higher doses may be used by specialist units.

Nausea and vomiting of terminal illness (where other drugs are unsuitable)
By mouth
- *Child 1–6 years*: 500 micrograms/kg every 4–6h; maximum 40mg daily.
- *Child 6–12 years*: 500 micrograms/kg every 4–6h; maximum 75mg daily.
- *Child 12–18 years*: 10–25mg every 4–6h.

By deep intramuscular injection
- *Child 1–6 years*: 500 micrograms/kg every 6–8h; maximum 40mg daily.
- *Child 6–12 years*: 500 micrograms/kg every 6–8h; maximum 75mg daily.
- *Child 12–18 years*: initially 25mg, then 25–50mg every 3–4h until vomiting stops.

Notes
- Not licensed in children for intractable hiccup.
- Caution in children with hepatic impairment (can precipitate coma), renal impairment (start with a small dose; increased cerebral sensitivity), cardiovascular disease, epilepsy (and conditions predisposing to epilepsy), depression, and myasthenia gravis.
- Caution is also required in severe respiratory disease and in children with a history of jaundice or who have blood dyscrasias (perform blood counts if unexplained infection or fever develops).
- Photosensitization may occur with higher dosages; children should avoid direct sunlight.
- Antipsychotic drugs may be contraindicated in CNS depression.

- Risk of contact sensitization; tablets should not be crushed, and solutions should be handled with care.
- Available as: tablets, coated (25mg, 50mg, 100mg); oral solution (25mg/5mL, 100mg/5mL); injection (25mg/mL in 1mL and 2mL ampoules).

Clobazam

Uses

- Adjunctive therapy for epilepsy.

Dose and routes

For oral administration

- *Child 1 month to 6 years*: initial dose of 125 micrograms/kg bd. Increase every 5 days, as necessary and as tolerated, to a usual maintenance dose of 250 micrograms/kg bd. Maximum dose 500 micrograms/kg (15mg single dose) bd.
- *Child 6–18 years*: initial dose of 5mg daily. Increase every 5 days, as necessary and as tolerated, to a usual maintenance dose of 0.3–1mg/kg daily. Maximum 60mg daily. Daily doses of up to 30mg may be given as a single dose at bedtime; higher doses should be divided.

Notes

- Not licensed for use in children <6 years of age.
- Once titrated to an effective dose of clobazam, patients should remain on their treatment, and care should be exercised when changing between different formulations.
- Tablets can be administered whole, or crushed and mixed in apple sauce. The 10mg tablets can be divided into equal halves of 5mg. Clobazam can be given with or without food.
- Possible side effects as would be expected from benzodiazepines. Children are more susceptible to sedation and paradoxical emotional reactions.
- Available as: tablets (10mg Frisium®), tablets (5mg—unlicensed and available on a named-patient basis), and oral liquid (5mg in 5mL and 10mg in 5mL—care with differing strengths).
- Frisium® tablets are NHS-blacklisted, except for epilepsy and endorsed 'SLS'.

Clonazepam

Uses

- Tonic–clonic seizures.
- Partial seizures.
- Cluster seizures.
- Myoclonus.
- Status epilepticus (third-line, particularly in neonates).
- Neuropathic pain.

- Restless legs.
- Gasping.
- Anxiety and panic.

Dose and routes

By mouth (anticonvulsant doses: reduce for other indications)

- *Child 1 month to 1 year*: initially 250 micrograms at night for four nights, increased over 2–4 weeks to usual maintenance dose of 0.5–1mg at night (may be given in three divided doses, if necessary).
- *Child 1–5 years*: initially 250 micrograms at night for four nights, increased over 2–4 weeks to usual maintenance of 1–3mg at night (may be given in three divided doses, if necessary).
- *Child 5–12 years*: initially 500 micrograms at night for four nights, increased over 2–4 weeks to usual maintenance dose of 3–6mg at night (may be given in three divided doses, if necessary).
- *Child 12–18 years*: initially 1mg at night for four nights, increased over 2–4 weeks to usual maintenance of 4–8mg at night (may be given in three divided doses, if necessary).

For status epilepticus

Continuous subcutaneous infusion

- *Child 1 month to 18 years*: starting dose 20–25 micrograms/kg/24h.
- Maximum starting doses: 1–5 years: 250 micrograms/24h; 5–12 years: 500 micrograms/24h.
- Increase at intervals of not less than 12h to 200 micrograms/kg/24h (maximum 8mg/24h).
- Doses of up to 1.4mg/kg/24h have been used in status epilepticus in PICU environment.

By intravenous injection over at least 2min, or infusion

- *Neonate*: 100 micrograms/kg iv over at least 2min, repeated after 24h if necessary (avoid unless no safer alternative). Used for seizures not controlled with phenobarbital or phenytoin.
- *Child 1 month to 12 years*: loading dose 50 micrograms/kg (maximum 1mg) by iv injection, followed by infusion of 10 micrograms/kg/h, adjusted according to response; maximum 60 micrograms/kg/h.
- *Child 12–18 years*: loading dose 1mg by iv injection, followed by iv infusion of 10 micrograms/kg/h, adjusted according to response; maximum 60 micrograms/kg/h.

Notes

- Licensed for use in children for status epilepticus and epilepsy. Not licensed for neuropathic pain. Tablets licensed in children.
- Very effective anticonvulsant, usually third-line due to side effects and development of tolerance.
- Use lower doses for panic, anxiolysis, terminal sedation, neuropathic pain, and restless legs.
- Do not use in acute or severe respiratory insufficiency, unless in the imminently dying. Be cautious in those with chronic respiratory disease.

- As an anxiolytic/sedative, clonazepam is ~20 times as potent as diazepam (i.e. 250 micrograms of clonazepam equivalent to 5mg of diazepam po).
- Multiple indications, in addition to anticonvulsant activity, can make clonazepam particularly useful in the palliative care of children for neurological disorders.
- Many children with complex seizure disorders are on bd doses and higher dosages.
- The dose may be increased for short periods of 3–5 days with increased seizures, e.g. from viral illness.
- Elimination half-life of 20–40h means that it may take up to 6 days to reach steady state; there is a risk of accumulation and toxicity with a rapid increase of infusion; consider a loading dose to reach steady state more quickly.
- Avoid abrupt withdrawal.
- Associated with salivary hypersecretion and drooling.
- Tablets may be dispersed in water for administration via an enteral feeding tube.
- Stability of diluted clonazepam is up to 12h, so prescribers should consider 12-hourly infusions.
- Compatible with most drugs commonly administered via CSCI via a syringe driver.
- Available as: tablets (500 micrograms scored, 2mg scored); liquid (0.5mg in 5mL and 2mg in 5mL now available as licensed preparations from Rosemont, but not indicated in children due to high alcohol content; other unlicensed oral liquids are available from specials manufacturers); injection (1mg/mL unlicensed).

Clonidine

Uses
- Anxiety/sedation (prior to procedure).
- Pain/sedation/opioid-sparing/prevention of opioid withdrawal effects.
- Regional nerve block.
- Spasticity.
- Behavioural symptoms of irritability, impulsiveness, aggression.

Doses and routes
Anxiety/sedation/pre-procedure

Oral/intranasal/rectal
- *Child >1 month*: 4 micrograms/kg as a single dose (suggested maximum 150 micrograms single dose). If used as premedicant prior to a procedure, give 45–60min before.

Pain/sedation/opioid-sparing/prevention of opioid withdrawal effects (most experienced on PICU)
Oral/intravenous bolus
- *Child >1 month*: initial dose 1 microgram/kg/dose 3–4 times daily. Increase gradually, as needed and tolerated, to a maximum of 5 micrograms/kg/dose qds.

Intravenous infusion
- *Child >1 month*: 0.1–2 micrograms/kg/h.
- Usual starting doses:
  - *child <6 months*: 0.4 micrograms/kg/h;
  - *child >6 months*: 0.6 micrograms/kg/h.

For chronic long-term pain, and once an effective oral dose has been established, consideration can be made to transferring to transdermal patches using a patch size that will give a roughly equivalent daily dose of clonidine (see **➜** Notes below).

Regional nerve block—only in situations where specialist input is available
- *Child >3 months*: 1–2 micrograms/kg of clonidine in combination with a local anaesthetic.

Spasticity/movement disorder
Oral
- *Child >1 month*: 1–5 micrograms/kg/dose tds. Frequency of dosing may need to be increased and/or alternative route of administration considered if the enteral route is not possible.

Behavioural problems/tics/Tourette's syndrome
Oral
- *Child >4 years*: oral—initial dose of 25 micrograms at night. Increase, as necessary, after 1–2 weeks to 50 micrograms at night. Dose can be further increased by 25 micrograms every 2 weeks to a suggested maximum of 5 micrograms/kg/day or 300 micrograms/day.

Notes
- Clonidine is a mixed alpha-1 and alpha-2 agonist (mainly alpha-2). Appears to have synergistic analgesic effects with opioids and prevent opioid withdrawal symptoms. Also useful for its sedative effect. Use established in attention-deficit/hyperactivity disorder (ADHD), behavioural problems, and tics.
- Not licensed for use in children.
- Licensed indication of clonidine is for the treatment of hypertension, so reduction in blood pressure (BP) is a likely side effect of use. Titrate the dose of clonidine against the symptoms, and monitor BP and pulse on starting treatment and after each dose increase.
- When used for longer than a few days, clonidine should be withdrawn slowly on discontinuation to prevent acute withdrawal symptoms, including rebound hypertension.
- Use with caution in those with bradyarrhythmia, Raynaud's, or other occlusive peripheral vascular disease.
- Common side effects include constipation, nausea, dry mouth, vomiting, postural hypotension, dizziness, sleep disturbances, headache.
- Effects of clonidine are abolished by drugs with alpha-2 antagonistic activity, e.g. tricyclics and antipsychotic drugs. Antihypertensive effects may be potentiated by other drugs used to lower BP.

- Oral bioavailability 75–100%; generally 1:1 conversion iv:oral is suggested as a starting point (largely adult data; note it has been suggested that oral bioavailability may be lower in children).
- Some reports of use of pr clonidine. Pharmacokinetic studies suggest almost 100% bioavailability via this route. Single pr doses of 2.5–4 micrograms/kg have been used.
- Onset of effect: oral 30–60min. Time to peak plasma concentration: oral 1.5–5h; epidural 20min; transdermal 2 days.
- Clonidine has been used successfully by sc injection and infusion—seek specialist advice.
- Oral solution may be administered via an enteral feeding tube. Alternatively, if the required dose is appropriate to the available tablet strengths, the tablets may be crushed and dispersed in water for administration via an enteral feeding tube. Note: the 25-micrograms tablets do not appear to disperse in water as readily as the 100-micrograms tablets.
- Chronic conditions—for older children, the use of transdermal patches may be considered when an effective oral dose has been established which is great enough to allow an approximate conversion (1:1) to the transdermal route. Although unlicensed in the UK, three strengths of patches are available, programmed to release 100 micrograms, 200 micrograms, or 300 micrograms of clonidine daily for 7 days.
- Available as: tablets 25 micrograms, 100 micrograms; injection 150 micrograms/mL; transdermal patch 100 micrograms, 200 micrograms, or 300 micrograms of clonidine daily for 7 days (not licensed in the UK—available via an importation company); and oral solution (special) 50 micrograms/mL.

Co-danthramer (dantron and poloxamer 188)

Uses
- Constipation in terminal illness only.

Dose and routes
By mouth

Co-danthramer 25/200 suspension 5mL = one co-danthramer 25/200 capsule (dantron 25mg, poloxamer '188' 200mg):
- *child 2–12 years*: 2.5–5mL at night;
- *child 6–12 years*: one capsule at night;
- *child 12–18 years*: 5–10mL or 1–2 capsules at night. Dosage can be increased up to 10–20mL bd.

Strong co-danthramer 75/1000 suspension 5mL = two strong co-danthramer 37.5/500 capsules:
- *child 12–18 years*: 5mL or 1–2 capsules at night.

Notes
- Co-danthramer is made from dantron and poloxamer '188'.
- Acts as a stimulant laxative.
- Avoid prolonged skin contact due to risk of irritation and excoriation (avoid in urinary or faecal incontinence/children with nappies).
- Dantron can turn urine red/brown.
- Rodent studies indicate potential carcinogenic risk.

Co-danthrusate (dantron and docusate sodium)

Uses
- Constipation in terminal illness only.

Dose and routes
By mouth
Co-danthrusate 50/60 suspension 5mL = one co-danthrusate 50/60 capsule (dantron 50mg/docusate sodium 60mg).
- *Child 6–12 years*: 5mL or one capsule at night.
- *Child 12–18 years*: 5–15mL or 1–3 capsules at night.

Notes
- Co-danthrusate is made from dantron and docusate sodium.
- Acts as a stimulant laxative.
- Avoid prolonged skin contact due to risk of irritation and excoriation (avoid in urinary or faecal incontinence/children with nappies).
- Danthron can turn urine red/brown.
- Rodent studies indicate potential carcinogenic risk.

Codeine phosphate

The EMA's Pharmacovigilance Risk Assessment Committee (PRAC) has addressed safety concerns with codeine-containing medicines when used for the management of pain in children (June 2013). This follows the PRAC's review of reports of children who developed serious adverse effects or died after taking codeine for pain relief. Children who are 'ultrarapid metabolizers' of codeine are at risk of severe opioid toxicity due to rapid and uncontrolled conversion of codeine into morphine.

The PRAC recommended the following risk minimization measures to ensure that only children for whom benefits are greater than the risks are given the medicine for pain relief:
- codeine-containing medicines should only be used to treat acute (short-lived) moderate pain in children above 12 years of age, and only if it cannot be relieved by other analgesics such as paracetamol or ibuprofen, because of the risk of respiratory depression associated with codeine use;

- codeine should not be used at all in children (aged below 18 years) with known obstructive airway disease or those who undergo surgery for the removal of the tonsils or adenoids to treat obstructive sleep apnoea, as these patients are more susceptible to respiratory problems.

(See ℘ http://www.ema.europa.eu/ema/index.jsp?curl=pages/news_and_events/news/2013/06/news_detail_001813.jsp&mid=WC0b01ac058004d5c1.)

Further, the WHO now advises there is insufficient evidence to make a recommendation for an alternative to codeine and recommends moving directly from non-opioids (step 1) to low-dose strong opioids for the management of moderate uncontrolled pain in children.

Uses

- Mild to moderate pain in patients who, through previous use, are known to be able to benefit when other agents are contraindicated or not appropriate. For when required use only—not suitable for management of background pain.
- Marked diarrhoea, when other agents are contraindicated or not appropriate, with medication doses and interval titrated to effect.
- Cough suppressant.

Dose and routes

By mouth, rectum, subcutaneous injection, or intramuscular injection

- *Neonate*: 0.5–1mg/kg every 4–6h.
- *Child 1 month to 12 years*: 0.5–1mg/kg every 4–6h; maximum 240mg daily.
- *Child 12–18 years*: 30–60mg every 4–6h; maximum 240mg daily.

As cough suppressant in the form of pholcodine linctus/syrup (NB. different strengths are available)

- *Child 6–12 years*: 2.5mg 3–4 times daily.
- *Child 12–18 years*: 5–10mg 3–4 times daily.

Notes

- Not licensed for use in children <1 year old.
- Codeine is effectively a prodrug for morphine, delivering ~1mg of morphine for every 10mg of codeine.
- Pharmacologically, codeine is no different from morphine, except that it is weaker and less consistently effective. This has led the WHO to recommend that it is better replaced by low doses of morphine.
- Conversion to morphine is subject to wide pharmacogenetic variation.
- 5–34% of population have an enzyme deficiency that prevents activation of codeine to the active metabolite, and so it is ineffective in this group.
- Individuals who are ultrarapid metabolizers can develop life-threatening opioid toxicity.
- Seems relatively constipating, compared with morphine/diamorphine, particularly in children.
- Rectal administration is an unlicensed route of administration using an unlicensed product.
- Must *not* be given iv.
- Reduce dose in renal impairment.

- Available as: tablets (15mg, 30mg, 60mg), oral solution (25mg/5mL), injection (60mg/mL), and suppositories of various strengths available from 'specials' manufacturers. Pholcodine as linctus 2mg/5mL, 5mg/5mL, and 10mg/5mL.
- Some community pharmacies do not stock codeine phosphate solution at 25mg/5mL. They usually do stock codeine phosphate linctus at 15mg/5mL, and this is worth enquiring of if a practitioner is working in the community and wishes to prescribe this medication. BE CAREFUL WITH DIFFERING STRENGTHS OF LIQUIDS.

Cyclizine

Uses
- Antiemetic of choice for raised intracranial pressure.
- Nausea and vomiting where other more specific antiemetics (metoclopramide, $5HT_3$ antagonists) have failed.

Dose and routes
By mouth or by slow intravenous injection over 3–5min
- *Child 1 month to 6 years*: 0.5–1mg/kg up to tds; maximum single dose 25mg.
- *Child 6–12 years*: 25mg up to tds.
- *Child 12–18 years*: 50mg up to tds.

By rectum
- *Child 2–6 years*: 12.5mg up to tds.
- *Child 6–12 years*: 25mg up to tds.
- *Child 12–18 years*: 50mg up to tds.

By continuous intravenous or subcutaneous infusion
- *Child 1 month to 5 years*: 3mg/kg over 24h (maximum 50mg/24h).
- *Child 6–12 years*: 75mg over 24h.
- *Child 12–18 years*: 150mg over 24h.

Notes
- Antihistaminic, antimuscarinic, antiemetic.
- Tablets are not licensed for use in children <6 years old.
- Injection is not licensed for use in children.
- Antimuscarinic side effects include dry mouth, drowsiness, headache, fatigue, dizziness, thickening of bronchial secretions, and nervousness.
- Rapid sc or iv bolus can lead to 'light-headedness'—disliked by some and enthralling to others, leading to repeated quests for iv cyclizine.
- Care with sc or iv infusion—acidic pH and can cause injection site reactions.
- For CSCI or iv infusion, dilute only with water for injection (WFI) or 5% glucose; *incompatible* with 0.9% saline and will precipitate.
- Concentration-dependent incompatibility with alfentanil, dexamethasone, diamorphine, and oxycodone.
- Suppositories must be kept refrigerated.

- Tablets may be crushed for oral administration. The tablets do not disperse well in water, but, if shaken in 10mL of water for 5min, the resulting dispersion may be administered immediately via an enteral feeding tube.
- Available as: tablets (50mg), suppositories (12.5mg, 25mg, 50mg, 100mg from 'specials' manufacturers), and injection (50mg/mL).

Dantrolene

Uses
- Skeletal muscle relaxant.
- Chronic severe muscle spasm or spasticity.

Dose and routes
The dose of dantrolene should be built up slowly.

By mouth
- *Child 5–12 years*: initial dose of 500 micrograms/kg once daily (od); after 7 days, increase to 500 micrograms/kg/dose tds. Every 7 days, increase by a further 500 micrograms/kg/dose until response. Maximum recommended dose is 2mg/kg 3–4 times daily (maximum total daily dose 400mg).
- *Child 12–18 years*: initial dose of 25mg od; after 7 days, increase to 25mg tds. Every 7 days, increase by a further 500 micrograms/kg/dose until response. Maximum recommended dose is 2mg/kg 3–4 times daily (maximum total daily dose 400mg).

Notes
- Not licensed for use in children.
- Hepatotoxicity risk; consider checking liver function before, and at regular intervals during, therapy. Contraindicated in hepatic impairment—avoid in liver disease or concomitant use of hepatotoxic drugs.
- Can cause drowsiness, dizziness, weakness, and diarrhoea.
- Available as: capsules (25mg, 100mg) and oral suspension (extemporaneous formulation).

Dexamethasone

Uses
- Headache associated with raised intracranial pressure caused by a tumour.
- Anti-inflammatory in the brain and other tumours causing pressure on nerves or bone, or obstruction of hollow viscus.
- Analgesic role in nerve compression, spinal cord compression, and bone pain.
- Antiemetic either as an adjuvant or in highly emetogenic cytotoxic therapies.

Dose and routes

Prescribe as a dexamethasone base.

Headache associated with raised intracranial pressure

By mouth or intravenously

- *Child 1 month to 12 years*: 250 micrograms/kg bd for 5 days; then reduce or stop.

To relieve symptoms of brain or other tumour

Numerous other indications in cancer management, such as spinal cord and/or nerve compression, some causes of dyspnoea, bone pain, SVC obstruction, etc.; only in discussion with the specialist palliative medicine team. High doses <16mg/24h may be advised.

Antiemetic

By mouth or intravenously

- *Child <1 year*: initial dose 250 micrograms tds. This dose may be increased, as necessary and as tolerated, up to 1mg tds.
- *Child 1–5 years*: initial dose 1mg tds. This dose may be increased, as necessary and as tolerated, up to 2mg tds.
- *Child 6–12 years*: initial dose 2mg tds. This dose may be increased, as necessary and as tolerated, up to 4mg tds.
- *Child 12–18 years*: 4mg tds.

Notes

- Not licensed for use in children as an antiemetic.
- Dexamethasone has high glucocorticoid activity, but insignificant mineralocorticoid activity, so is particularly suited for high-dose anti-inflammatory therapy.
- Dexamethasone can be given in a single daily dose each morning for most indications; this reduces the likelihood of corticosteroid-induced insomnia and agitation.
- Dexamethasone has an oral bioavailability of >80%; it can be converted to sc or iv on a 1:1 basis.
- Dexamethasone 1mg = dexamethasone phosphate 1.2mg = dexamethasone sodium phosphate 1.3mg.
- Dexamethasone 1mg = 7mg prednisolone (anti-inflammatory equivalence).
- Dexamethasone has a long duration of action.
- Problems of weight gain and Cushingoid appearance are major problems specifically in children. All specialist units therefore use pulsed-dose regimes, in preference to continual use. Regimes vary with conditions and specialist units. Seek local specialist advice.
- Other side effects include: diabetes, osteoporosis, muscle wasting, peptic ulceration, and behavioural problems, particularly agitation.
- Dexamethasone can be stopped abruptly if given for a short duration of time (<7 days); otherwise gradual withdrawal is advised.
- Tablets may be dispersed in water if oral liquid unavailable. Oral solution or tablets dispersed in water may be administered via an enteral feeding tube.

- Available as: tablets (500 micrograms, 2mg), oral solution (2mg/5mL and other strengths available from 'specials' manufacturers), and injection as dexamethasone sodium phosphate (equivalent to 4mg/1mL dexamethasone base (Organon® brand) or 3.3mg/mL dexamethasone base (Hospira® brand)).

Diamorphine

Uses
- Moderate to severe pain.
- Dyspnoea.

Dose and routes
Normally convert using OME from previous analgesia.

Use the following *starting* doses in opioid-naïve patients. The maximum dose stated applies to the *starting* dose only.

Acute or chronic pain
By continuous subcutaneous or intravenous infusion
- Neonate: initial dose of 2.5 micrograms/kg/h which can be increased, as necessary, to a suggested maximum of 7 micrograms/kg/h.
- Child 1 month to 18 years: 7–25 micrograms/kg/h (initial maximum 10mg/24h), adjusted according to response.

By intravenous, subcutaneous, or intramuscular injection
- Neonate: 15 micrograms/kg every 6h, as necessary, adjusted according to response.
- Child 1–3 months: 20 micrograms/kg every 6h, as necessary, adjusted according to response.
- Child 3–6 months: 25–50 micrograms/kg every 6h, as necessary, adjusted according to response.
- Child 6–12 months: 75 micrograms/kg every 4h, as necessary, adjusted according to response.
- Child 1–12 years: 75–100 micrograms/kg every 4h, as necessary, adjusted according to response. Suggested initial maximum dose of 2.5mg.
- Child 12–18 years: 75–100 micrograms/kg every 4h, as necessary, adjusted according to response. Suggested initial maximum dose of 2.5–5mg.

By intranasal or buccal route
- Child over 10kg: 50–100 micrograms/kg; maximum single dose 10mg.

Injection solution can be used by intranasal or buccal routes or a nasal spray (Ayendi®) now available and licensed for use in children aged 2 years and over (weight 12kg upwards) for the management of severe acute pain.

720 micrograms/actuation
- 12–18kg: two sprays as a single dose.
- 18–24kg: three sprays as a single dose.
- 24–30kg: four sprays as a single dose.

1600 micrograms/actuation
- 30–40kg: two sprays as a single dose.
- 40–50kg: three sprays as a single dose.

Breakthrough

By buccal, subcutaneous, or intravenous routes
- For breakthrough pain, use 5–10% of total daily diamorphine dose every 1–4h, as needed.

Dyspnoea

By buccal, subcutaneous, or intravenous routes
- Dose as for pain, but at 50% of breakthrough dose.

Notes

- Diamorphine injection is licensed for the treatment of children who are terminally ill.
- For intranasal or buccal administration of diamorphine, use the injection powder reconstituted in WFIs (unlicensed route of administration), or the nasal spray may be used (licensed for use in the management of severe acute pain from 2 years of age).
- In neonates, the dosage interval should be extended to 6- or 8-hourly, depending on renal function, and the dose carefully checked, due to increased sensitivity to opioids in the first year of life.
- In poor renal function, the dosage interval may be lengthened, or opioids only given as required and titrated against symptoms. Consider changing to fentanyl.
- For CSCI, dilute with WFIs, as concentration incompatibility occurs with 0.9% saline at above 40mg/mL.
- Diamorphine can be given by sc infusion up to a strength of 250mg/mL.
- Morphine injection is rapidly taking over from diamorphine, as the only benefit of diamorphine over morphine is its better solubility when high doses are needed, and this is rarely a problem in paediatric doses.
- Available as: injection (5mg, 10mg, 30mg, 100mg, 500mg ampoules) and nasal spray 720 micrograms/actuation and 1600 micrograms/actuation (Ayendi® nasal spray).

Diazepam

Uses

- Short-term anxiety relief.
- Agitation.
- Panic attacks.
- Relief of muscle spasm.
- Treatment of status epilepticus.

Dose and routes

Short-term anxiety relief, panic attacks, and agitation

By mouth
- *Child 2–12 years*: 1–2mg tds.
- *Child 12–18 years*: initial dose of 2mg tds, increasing, as necessary and as tolerated, to a maximum of 10mg tds.

Relief of muscle spasm

By mouth
- *Child 1–12 months*: initial dose of 250 micrograms/kg bd.
- *Child 1–5 years*: initial dose of 2.5mg bd.
- *Child 5–12 years*: initial dose of 5mg bd.
- *Child 12–18 years*: initial dose of 10mg bd; maximum total daily dose 40mg.

Status epilepticus

By intravenous injection over 3–5min
- *Neonate*: 300–400 micrograms/kg as a single dose, repeated once after 10min, if necessary.
- *Child 1 month to 12 years*: 300–400 micrograms/kg (maximum 10mg), repeated once after 10min, if necessary.
- *Child 12–18 years*: 10mg, repeated once after 10min, if necessary (in hospital, up to 20mg as a single dose may be used).

By rectum (rectal solution)
- *Neonate*: 1.25–2.5mg, repeated once after 10min, if necessary.
- *Child 1 month to 2 years*: 5mg, repeated once after 10min, if necessary.
- *Child 2–12 years*: 5–10mg, repeated once after 10min, if necessary.
- *Child 12–18 years*: 10mg, repeated once after 10min, if necessary (in hospital, up to 20mg as a single dose may be used).

Notes
- Do not use in acute or severe respiratory insufficiency, unless in the imminently dying.
- Rectal tubes not licensed for children <1 year old.
- Use with caution in mild to moderate hepatic disease.
- Metabolized via the cytochrome P450 group of liver enzymes—potential for interaction with any concurrent medicine that induces or inhibits this group of enzymes. Enhancement of the central depressive effect may occur if diazepam is combined with drugs such as neuroleptics, antipsychotics, tranquillizers, antidepressants, hypnotics, analgesics, anaesthetics, barbiturates, and sedative antihistamines.
- Can cause dose-dependent drowsiness and impaired psychomotor and cognitive skills.
- Almost 100% bioavailable when given po or by rectal solution.
- Onset of action ~15min given po and within 1–5min given iv. Given as rectal solution, diazepam is rapidly absorbed from the rectal mucosa, with maximum serum concentration reached within 17min.
- Long plasma half-life of 24–48h, with the active metabolite nordiazepam having a plasma half-life of 48–120h.
- The oral solution may be administered via a gastrostomy tube. For administration via a jejunostomy tube, consider using tablets dispersed in water to reduce osmolarity.
- Available as: tablets (2mg, 5mg, 10mg), oral solution (2mg/5mL, 5mg/5mL), rectal tubes (2.5mg, 5mg, 10mg), and injection (5mg/mL solution and 5mg/mL emulsion).

Diclofenac sodium

Uses
- Mild to moderate pain and inflammation, particularly musculoskeletal disorders.

Dose and routes
By mouth or rectum
- *Child 6 months to 18 years*: initial dose of 0.3mg/kg tds, increasing, if necessary, to a maximum of 1mg/kg tds (maximum 50mg single dose).

By intramuscular or intravenous infusion
- *Child 2–18 years*: initial dose of 0.3mg/kg 1–2 times daily; maximum of 150mg/day and for a maximum of 2 days.

Notes
Will cause closure of ductus arteriosus; contraindicated in duct-dependent congenital heart disease.
- Not licensed for use in children under 1 year; *suppositories* not licensed for use in children under 6 years, except for use in children over 1 year for juvenile idiopathic arthritis; solid dose forms containing >25mg not licensed for use in children; *injection (for im bolus or iv infusion only)* not licensed for use in children.
- The risk of cardiovascular events secondary to NSAID use is undetermined in children. In adults, all NSAID use (including COX-2 selective inhibitors) can, to varying degrees, be associated with a small increased risk of thrombotic events (e.g. myocardial infarction and stroke), independent of baseline cardiovascular risk factors or duration of NSAID use; however, the greatest risk may be in those patients receiving high doses long-term. A small increased thrombotic risk cannot be excluded in children.
- All NSAIDs are associated with gastrointestinal toxicity. In adults, evidence on the relative safety of NSAIDs indicates differences in the risks of serious upper gastrointestinal side effects—piroxicam and ketorolac are associated with the highest risk; indometacin, diclofenac, and naproxen are associated with intermediate risk, and ibuprofen with the lowest risk (although high doses of ibuprofen have been associated with intermediate risk).
- The smallest dose that can be given practically by the rectal route is 3.125mg by cutting a 12.5mg suppository into quarters (CC).
- For iv infusion, dilute in 5% glucose or 0.9% NaCl, and infuse over 30–120min.
- Dispersible tablets may be administered via an enteral feeding tube. Disperse immediately before administration.
- Available as: tablets (25mg, 50mg, and 75mg modified-release), dispersible tablets (10mg from a 'specials' manufacturer, 50mg), modified-release capsules (75mg and 100mg), injection (25mg/mL Voltarol® for im injection or iv infusion only), and suppositories (12.5mg, 25mg, 50mg, and 100mg).

Dihydrocodeine

Uses
- Mild to moderate pain in patients known to be able to benefit.

Dose and routes
By mouth or deep subcutaneous or intramuscular injection
- *Child 1–4 years*: 500 micrograms/kg every 4–6h.
- *Child 4–12 years*: initial dose of 500 micrograms/kg (maximum 30mg/ dose) every 4–6h. Dose may be increased, if necessary, to 1mg/kg every 4–6h (maximum 30mg/dose).
- *Child 12–18 years*: 30mg (maximum 50mg by im or deep sc injection) every 4–6h.
- Modified-release tablets used 12-hourly (use half of previous total daily dose for each modified-release dose).

Notes
- Most preparations not licensed for children under 4 years.
- Relatively constipating, compared with morphine/diamorphine, and has a ceiling analgesic effect.
- Dihydrocodeine is itself an active substance, not a prodrug like codeine.
- Oral bioavailability 20%, so probably equipotent with codeine by mouth (but opinion varies), twice as potent as codeine by injection.
- Time to onset 30min; duration of action 4h for immediate-release tablets.
- Side effects as for other opioids, plus paralytic ileus, abdominal pain, and paraesthesiae.
- Precautions: avoid or reduce dose in hepatic or renal failure.
- Available as: tablets (30mg, 40mg), oral solution (10mg/5mL), injection (CD) (50mg/mL 1mL ampoules), and modified-release tablets (60mg, 90mg, 120mg).

Docusate

Uses
- Constipation (faecal softener).

Dose and routes
By mouth
- *Child 6 months to 2 years*: initial dose of 12.5mg tds; adjust dose, according to response.
- *Child 2–12 years*: initial dose of 12.5mg tds. Increase to 25mg tds, as necessary, and then further adjust dose, according to response.
- *Child 12–18 years*: initial dose 100mg/dose tds. Adjust as needed, according to response, up to 500mg/day in divided doses.

By rectum
- *Child 12–18 years*: one enema as a single dose.

Notes

- Adult oral solution and capsules not licensed in children <12 years.
- Oral preparations act within 1–2 days.
- Rectal preparations act within 20min.
- Mechanism of action is emulsifying, wetting, and mild stimulant.
- Doses may be exceeded on specialist advice.
- Available as: capsules (100mg), oral solution (12.5mg/5mL paediatric, 50mg/5mL adult), and enema (120mg in 10g single-dose pack).

Domperidone

Medicines and Healthcare products Regulatory Agency (MHRA), April 2014: domperidone is associated with a small increased risk of serious cardiac side effects. Its use is now restricted to the relief of symptoms of nausea and vomiting, and the dosage and duration of use have been reduced. Domperidone is now *contraindicated* for use in those with underlying cardiac conditions and other risk factors.

The indications and doses below are therefore largely unlicensed usage in a particular population. Use the minimum effective dose. Do not use in those with known cardiac problems or other risk factors.

Uses

- Nausea and vomiting where poor gastrointestinal motility is the cause.
- Gastro-oesophageal reflux resistant to other therapy.

Dose and routes

For nausea and vomiting

By mouth

- *>1 month and body weight ≤35kg*: initial dose of 250 micrograms/kg 3–4 times daily, increasing, if necessary, to 500 micrograms/kg 3–4 times daily. Maximum 2.4mg/kg (or 80mg) in 24h.
- *Body weight >35kg*: initial dose of 10mg 3–4 times daily, increasing, if necessary, to 20mg 3–4 times daily. Maximum 80mg in 24h.

By rectum

- *Body weight 15–35kg*: 30mg bd.
- *Body weight >35kg*: 60mg bd.

For gastro-oesophageal reflux and gastrointestinal stasis

By mouth

- *Neonate*: initial dose of 100 micrograms/kg 4–6 times daily before feeds. Dose may be increased, if necessary, to maximum of 300 micrograms/kg 4–6 times daily.
- *Child 1 month to 12 years*: initial dose of 200 micrograms/kg (maximum single dose 10mg) 3–4 times daily before food. Dose may be increased, if necessary, to 400 micrograms/kg 3–4 times daily. Maximum single dose 20mg.
- *Child 12–18 years*: initial dose of 10mg 3–4 times daily before food. Dose may be increased, if necessary, to 20mg 3–4 times daily.

Notes

- Domperidone may be associated with an increased risk of serious ventricular arrhythmias or sudden cardiac death.
- Domperidone is contraindicated in those:
  - with conditions where cardiac conduction is, or could be, impaired;
  - with underlying cardiac diseases such as congestive heart failure;
  - receiving other medications known to prolong the QT interval (e.g. erythromycin, ketoconazole) or which are potent CYP3A4 inhibitors;
  - with severe hepatic impairment.
- This risk may be higher with daily doses >30mg. Use at the lowest effective dose.
- Not licensed for use in gastrointestinal stasis; not licensed for use in children for GORD.
- Reduced ability to cross the blood–brain barrier, so less likely to cause extrapyramidal side effects, compared with metoclopramide.
- Promotes gastrointestinal motility, so diarrhoea can be an unwanted (or useful) side effect.
- Not to be used in patients with hepatic impairment.
- For administration via an enteral feeding tube—use the suspension formulation, although the total daily dose of sorbitol should be considered. If administering into the jejunum, dilute the suspension with at least an equal volume of water immediately prior to administration.
- Available as: tablets (10mg), oral suspension (5mg/5mL), and suppositories (30mg).

Entonox® (nitrous oxide)

Uses

- As self-regulated analgesia, without loss of consciousness.
- Particularly useful for painful dressing changes.

Dose and routes

By inhalation

- *Child usually >5 years old*: self-administration using a demand valve. Up to 50% in oxygen, according to the child's needs.

Notes

- Is normally used as a light anaesthesic.
- Rapid onset and then offset.
- Should only be used as self-administration, using a demand valve; all other situations require a specialist paediatric anaesthetist.
- Use is dangerous in the presence of pneumothorax or intracranial air after head injury.
- Prolonged use can cause megaloblastic anaemia.
- May be difficult to make available in hospice settings, especially if needed infrequently, due to training, governance, and supply implications.

Erythromycin

Uses
• Gastrointestinal stasis (motilin receptor agonist).

Dose and routes
By mouth
• *Neonate*: 3mg/kg qds.
• *Child 1 month to 18 years*: 3mg/kg qds.

Notes
• Not licensed for use in children with gastrointestinal stasis.
• Erythromycin is excreted principally by the liver, so caution should be exercised in administering the antibiotic to patients with impaired hepatic function or concomitantly receiving potentially hepatotoxic agents.
• Erythromycin is a known inhibitor of the cytochrome P450 system and may increase the serum concentration of drugs which are metabolized by this system. Appropriate monitoring should be undertaken, and dosage should be adjusted, as necessary. Particular care should be taken with medications known to prolong the QT interval of the electrocardiogram (ECG).
• Available as: tablets (250mg, 500mg) and oral suspension (125mg/5mL, 250mg/5mL, 500mg/5mL).

Etamsylate

Uses
• Treatment of haemorrhage, including surface bleeding from ulcerating tumours.

Dose and routes
By mouth
• *>18 years*: 500mg qds, indefinitely or until a week after cessation of bleeding.

Notes
• Not licensed for use in children with haemorrhage.
• Available as: tablets (500mg).

Etoricoxib

Uses
- Anti-inflammatory analgesic; adjuvant for musculoskeletal pain.

Dose and routes
Oral
- *Child 12–16 years*: initial dose of 30mg od. Dose may be increased, as necessary and as tolerated, to a maximum of 60mg od.
- *Child 16 years and older*: usual dose of 30–90mg od. Doses up to 120mg have been used on a short-term basis in acute gouty arthritis in adults.

Notes
- Oral selective COX-2 inhibitor.
- Etoricoxib is not licensed for use in children <16 years of age. The pharmacokinetics of etoricoxib in children <12 years of age have not been studied.
- Etoricoxib may mask fever and other signs of inflammation.
- All NSAIDs should be used with caution in children with a history of hypersensitivity to any NSAID or in those with a coagulation disorder.
- Etoricoxib is contraindicated in those with: active peptic ulceration or active gastrointestinal bleeding, severe hepatic or renal dysfunction, inflammatory bowel disease, or congestive heart failure.
- The risk of cardiovascular events secondary to NSAID use is undetermined in children. In adults, COX-2 selective inhibitors, diclofenac (150mg daily), and ibuprofen (2.4g daily) are associated with an increased risk of thrombotic effects (e.g. myocardial infarction and stroke).
- All NSAIDs are associated with gastrointestinal toxicity. In adults, evidence on the relative safety of NSAIDs indicates differences in the risks of serious upper gastrointestinal side effects, with piroxicam and ketorolac associated with the highest risk, and ibuprofen at low to medium dose with the lowest risk. Selective COX-2 inhibitors are associated with a lower risk of serious upper gastrointestinal side effects than non-selective NSAIDs. Children appear to tolerate NSAIDs better than adults, and gastrointestinal side effects are less common, although they do still occur.
- Common (1–10% of patients) adverse events: alveolar osteitis; oedema/fluid retention; dizziness, headache; palpitations, arrhythmia; hypertension; bronchospasm; abdominal pain; constipation, flatulence, gastritis, heartburn/acid reflux, diarrhoea, dyspepsia/epigastric discomfort, nausea, vomiting, oesophagitis, oral ulcer; alanine aminotransferase (ALT) increased, aspartate aminotransferase (AST) increased; ecchymosis; asthenia/fatigue, flu-like disease.
- Potential drug interactions include warfarin (increase in international normalized ratio (INR)), and diuretics, angiotensin-converting enzyme (ACE) inhibitors, and angiotensin II antagonists (increased risk of compromised renal function). Etoricoxib does NOT appear to inhibit or induce CYP isoenzymes. However, the main pathway of etoricoxib

metabolism is dependent on CYP enzymes (primarily CYP3A4), so co-administration with drugs that are inducers or inhibitors of this pathway may affect the metabolism of etoricoxib.

- Etoricoxib is administered po and may be taken with or without food. However, the onset of effect may be faster when administered without food.
- Etoricoxib tablets may be dispersed in 10mL of water and will disintegrate to give fine granules that settle quickly but disperse easily and flush down an 8Fr NG or gastrostomy tube without blockage.
- Available as: film-coated tablets (30mg, 60mg, 90mg, 120mg). Tablets contain lactose.

Fentanyl

Uses
- Step 2 WHO pain ladder, once dose is titrated.

Dose and routes
Normally convert using OME from previous analgesia.

Use the following *starting* doses in the opioid-naïve patient. The maximum dose stated applies to the *starting* dose only.

By transmucosal application (lozenge with oromucosal applicator)
- Child 2–18 years and >10kg: 15 micrograms/kg as a single dose, titrated to a maximum dose of 400 micrograms (higher doses under specialist supervision).

By intranasal
- Neonate to child <2 years: 1 microgram/kg as a single dose.
- Child 2–18 years: 1–2 micrograms/kg as a single dose, with an initial maximum single dose of 50 micrograms.

By transdermal patch or continuous infusion
- Based on oral morphine dose equivalent (given as 24h totals).

By intravenous injection
- Neonate or infant: 1–2 micrograms/kg per dose slowly over 3–5min; repeated every 2–4h.
- Child: 1–2 micrograms/kg per dose; repeated every 30–60min.

By continuous intravenous infusion
- Neonate or infant: initial iv bolus of 1–2 micrograms/kg (slowly over 3–5min), followed by 0.5–1 micrograms/kg/h.
- Child: initial iv bolus of 1–2 micrograms/kg (slowly over 3–5min), followed by 0.5–1 micrograms/kg/h.

The 72h fentanyl patches are *approximately* equivalent to the following 24h doses of oral morphine.

Morphine salt 30mg daily	≡	fentanyl '12' patch
Morphine salt 60mg daily	≡	fentanyl '25' patch
Morphine salt 120mg daily	≡	fentanyl '50' patch
Morphine salt 180mg daily	≡	fentanyl '75' patch
Morphine salt 240mg daily	≡	fentanyl '100' patch

Notes

- Fentanyl patches should be changed every 72h, and the site of application rotated.
- Injection not licensed for use in children <2 years of age. Lozenges and nasal sprays are not licensed for use in children.
- The injection solution can be administered by the intranasal route for doses <50 micrograms which is the lowest strength of nasal spray available.
- Injection solution could be administered drop-wise (may be unpleasant) or using an atomizer device that Accident and Emergency units use for intranasal diamorphine.
- The main advantage of fentanyl over morphine in children is its availability as a transdermal formulation.
- It can simplify analgesic management in patients with poor, deteriorating, or even absent renal function.
- Avoid or reduce dose in hepatic impairment.
- It is a synthetic opioid, very different in structure from morphine, and therefore ideal for opioid switching.
- Evidence that it is less constipating than morphine has not been confirmed in more recent studies.
- The patch formulation is not usually suitable for the initiation or titration phases of opioid management in palliative care, since the patches represent large increments and because of the time lag to achieve steady state.
- The usefulness of lozenges in children is limited by the dose availability and no reliable conversion factor which also varies between preparations. Another caution is that opioid morphine approximate equivalence of the smallest lozenge (200 micrograms) is 30mg, meaning it is probably suitable to treat breakthrough pain only for children receiving a total daily dose equivalent of 180mg morphine or more. Older children will often choose to remove the lozenge before it is completely dissolved, giving them some much valued control over their analgesia. NB. The lozenge must be rotated in the buccal pouch, and not sucked. Unsuitable for pain in advanced neuromuscular disorders where independent physical rotation of the lozenge is not possible.
- Pharmacokinetics of fentanyl intranasally are favourable, but it is not always practical and/or well tolerated in children.

Available as fentanyl citrate:
- intranasal spray (50 micrograms/metered spray, 100 micrograms/ metered spray, 200 micrograms/metered spray Instanyl®). Also available as PecFent® 100 micrograms/metered spray and 400 micrograms/ metered spray;
- lozenge with oromucosal applicator (200 micrograms, 400 micrograms, 600 micrograms, 800 micrograms, 1.2mg, 1.6mg Actiq®);
- sublingual tablets (100, 200, 300, 400, 600, and 800 micrograms Abstral®) and buccal tablets (Effentora® 100, 200, 400, 600, and 800 micrograms; Breakyl® 200, 400, 600, 800, and 1200 micrograms);
- patches (12 micrograms/h, 25 micrograms/h, 50 micrograms/h, 75 micrograms/h, 100 micrograms/h).

Fluconazole

Uses
- Mucosal candidiasis infection, invasive candidal infections, or prevention of fungal infections in immunocompromised patients.

Dose and routes
Mucosal candidal infection

By mouth or intravenous infusion
- *Neonate under 2 weeks*: 3–6mg/kg on the first day, then 3mg/kg every 72h.
- *Neonate between 2 and 4 weeks*: 3–6mg/kg on the first day, then 3mg/kg every 48h.
- *Child 1 month to 12 years*: 3–6mg/kg on the first day, then 3mg/kg (maximum 100mg) daily.
- *Child 12–18 years*: 50mg/day. Increase to 100mg/day in difficult infections.

Invasive candidal and cryptococcal infections

By mouth or intravenous infusion
- *Neonate under 2 weeks*: 6–12mg/kg every 72h.
- *Neonate over 2 weeks*: 6–12mg/kg every 48h.
- *Child 1 month to 18 years*: 6–12mg/kg (maximum 800mg) every 24h.

Prevention of fungal infections in immunocompromised patients

By mouth or intravenous infusion
- *Neonate under 2 weeks*: 3–12mg/kg every 72h.
- *Neonate over 2 weeks*: 3–12mg/kg every 48h.
- *Child 1 month to 18 years*: 3–12mg/kg (maximum 400mg) every 24h.

Notes
- Use for 7–14 days in oropharyngeal candidiasis.
- Use for 14–30 days in other mucosal infections.
- Different duration of use in severely immunocompromised patients.

- Fluconazole is a potent CYP2C9 inhibitor and a moderate CYP3A4 inhibitor. Fluconazole is also an inhibitor of CYP2C19. Fluconazole-treated patients who are concomitantly treated with medicinal products with a narrow therapeutic window metabolized through CYP2C9, CYP2C19, and CYP3A4 should be monitored.
- The most frequently (>1 in 10) reported adverse reactions are headache, abdominal pain, diarrhoea, nausea, vomiting, ALT increase, AST increase, blood alkaline phosphatase increase, and rash.
- For iv infusion, give over 10–30min; do not exceed an infusion rate of 5–10mL/min.
- Oral suspension may be administered via an enteral feeding tube.
- Available as: capsules (50mg, 150mg, 200mg), oral suspension (50mg/5mL, 200mg/mL), and iv infusion (2mg/mL in 2mL, 50mL or 100mL infusion bags).

Fluoxetine

Uses
- Major depression.

Dose and routes

By mouth
- *Child 8–18 years*: initial dose 10mg od. May increase after 1–2 weeks, if necessary, to a maximum of 20mg od.

Notes
- Licensed for use in children from 8 years of age.
- Use with caution in children, ideally with specialist psychiatric advice.
- Increased risk of anxiety for the first 2 weeks.
- Onset of benefit 3–4 weeks.
- Consider long half-life when adjusting dosage. Do not discontinue abruptly.
- May also help for neuropathic pain and intractable cough.
- Suicide-related behaviours have been more frequently observed in clinical trials amongst children and adolescents treated with antidepressants, compared with placebo. Mania and hypomania have been commonly reported in paediatric trials.
- The most commonly reported adverse reactions in patients treated with fluoxetine were headache, nausea, insomnia, fatigue, and diarrhoea. Undesirable effects may decrease in intensity and frequency with continued treatment and do not generally lead to cessation of therapy.
- Because the metabolism of fluoxetine (like tricyclic antidepressants and other selective serotonin antidepressants) involves the hepatic cytochrome CYP2D6 isoenzyme system, concomitant therapy with drugs also metabolized by this enzyme system may lead to drug interactions.
- Must not be used in combination with a MAOI.
- Available as: capsules (20mg) and oral liquid (20mg/5mL).

Gabapentin

Uses
- Adjuvant in neuropathic pain.

Dose and routes
By mouth

Child >2 years
- Day 1: 10mg/kg as a single dose (maximum single dose 300mg).
- Day 2: 10mg/kg bd (maximum single dose 300mg).
- Day 3 onwards: 10mg/kg tds (maximum single dose 300mg).
- Increase further, if necessary, to maximum of 20mg/kg/dose (maximum single dose 600mg).

From 12 years
- The maximum daily dose can be increased, according to response, to a maximum of 3600mg/day.

Notes
- Not licensed for use in children with neuropathic pain.
- Speed of titration after the first 3 days varies between increases every 3 days for fast regime to increases every 1–2 weeks in debilitated children or when on other CNS depressants.
- No consensus on dose for neuropathic pain. Doses given, based on doses for partial seizures and authors' experience.
- Dose reduction required in renal impairment. Consult the manufacturer's literature.
- Very common (>1 in 10) side effects: somnolence, dizziness, ataxia, viral infection, fatigue, fever.
- Capsules can be opened but have a bitter taste.
- Available as: capsules (100mg, 300mg, 400mg), tablets (600mg, 800mg), and oral solution 50mg in 5mL (Rosemont—however, this product contains propylene glycol, acesulfame K, and saccharin sodium, and levels may exceed the recommended WHO daily intake limits if high doses are given to adolescents with low body weight (39–50kg)).

Gaviscon®

Uses
- Gastro-oesophageal reflux, dyspepsia, and heartburn.

Dose and routes
By mouth
- *Neonate to 2 years, body weight <4.5kg*: one dose (half dual sachet) when required, mixed with feeds or with water for breastfed babies; maximum six doses in 24h.
- *Neonate to 2 years body weight >4.5kg*: two doses (one dual sachet) when required, mixed with feeds or with water for breastfed babies or older infants; maximum six doses in 24h.

Gaviscon®
- *Child 2–12 years*: one tablet or 5–10mL of liquid after meals and at bedtime.
- *Child 12–18 years*: 1–2 tablets or 10–20mL after meals and at bedtime.

Gaviscon® Advance
- *Child 2–12 years*: one tablet or 2.5–5mL after meals and at bedtime (under medical advice only).
- *Child 12–18 years*: 1–2 tablets or 5–10mL suspension after meals and at bedtime.

Notes
- Gaviscon Infant® sachets licensed for infants and young children up to 2 years of age, but use in <1 year only under medical supervision. Gaviscon® liquid and tablets—licensed for use from 2 years of age, but age 2–6 years only on medical advice. Gaviscon® Advance suspension and tablets licensed for use from 12 years of age; under 12 years on medical advice only.
- Gaviscon Infant® should not be used with feed thickeners nor with excessive fluid losses (e.g. fever, diarrhoea, vomiting).
- Gaviscon® liquid contains 3.1mmol of sodium per 5mL; Gaviscon® tablets contain 2.65mmol of sodium and also contain aspartame. Gaviscon® Advance suspension contains 2.3mmol of sodium and 1mmol of potassium per 5mL and 2.25mmol of sodium and 1mmol of potassium per 5mL and also contain aspartame. Gaviscon Infant® sachets contain 0.92mmol of sodium per dose (half dual sachet).
- Available as: Gaviscon® liquid and tablets, Gaviscon® Advance suspension and tablets, and infant sachets (come as dual sachets; each half of a dual sachet is considered one dose).

Glycerin (glycerol)

Uses
- Constipation.

Dose and routes
By rectum
- *Neonate*: tip of a glycerin suppository (slice a small chip of a 1g suppository with a blade).
- *Child 1 month to 1 year*: 1g infant suppository, as required.
- *Child 1–12 years*: 2g child suppository, as required.
- *Child 12–18 years*: 4g adult suppository, as required.

Notes
- Moisten with water before insertion.
- Hygroscopic and lubricant actions. May also be a rectal stimulant.
- Response usually in 20min to 3h.
- Available as: suppositories (1g, 2g, and 4g).

Glycopyrronium bromide

Uses
- Control of upper airways secretion and hypersalivation.

Dose and routes
By mouth
- *Child 1 month to 18 years*: initial dose of 40 micrograms/kg 3–4 times daily. The dose may be increased, as necessary, to 100 micrograms/kg 3–4 times daily. Maximum 2mg/dose given tds.

Subcutaneous
- *Child 1 month to 12 years*: initial dose of 4 micrograms/kg 3–4 times daily. The dose may be increased, as necessary, to 10 micrograms/kg 3–4 times daily. Maximum 200 micrograms/dose given qds.
- *Child 12–18 years*: 200 micrograms every 4h when required.

Continuous subcutaneous infusion
- *Child 1 month to 12 years*: initial dose of 10 micrograms/kg/24h. The dose may be increased, as necessary, to 40 micrograms/kg/24h (maximum 1.2mg/24h).
- *Child 12–18 years*: initial dose of 600 micrograms/24h. The dose may be increased, as necessary, to 1.2mg/24h. Maximum recommended dose is 2.4mg/24h.

Notes
- Not licensed for use in children for control of upper airways secretion and hypersalivation.
- Excessive secretions can cause distress to the child but more often cause distress to those around him.
- Treatment is more effective if started before secretions become too much of a problem.
- Glycopyrronium does not cross the blood–brain barrier and therefore has fewer side effects than hyoscine hydrobromide, which is also used for this purpose. Also fewer cardiac side effects.
- Slower-onset response than with hyoscine hydrobromide or butylbromide.
- Oral absorption of glycopyrronium is very poor, with wide inter-individual variation.
- For oral administration, injection solution may be given, or the tablets may be crushed and suspended in water. For administration via an enteral feeding tube, tablets may be dispersed in water. However, the coarse dispersion settles quickly. Flush the syringe and tube well to ensure all the dose is received.
- Administration by CSCI: good compatibility data available with other commonly used palliative agents.
- Available as: tablets (1mg and 2mg via an importation company, as the tablets are not licensed in the UK)—dosing often too inflexible for children and costly, and can be difficult to obtain; injection (200 micrograms/mL 1mL ampoules) can also be used po (unlicensed route); oral solution can also be prepared extemporaneously from glycopyrronium powder and obtained from a 'specials' manufacturer.

Haloperidol

Uses

- Nausea and vomiting where the cause is metabolic or in difficult-to-manage cases such as end-stage renal failure.
- Restlessness and confusion.
- Intractable hiccups.
- Psychosis, hallucination.

Dose and routes

By mouth for nausea and vomiting

- *Child 1 month to 12 years*: initial dose of 50 micrograms/kg/24h (initial maximum 3mg/24h) in divided doses. The dose may be increased, as necessary, to a maximum of 170 micrograms/kg/24h in divided doses.
- *Child 12–18 years*: 1.5mg od at night, increasing, as necessary, to 1.5mg bd; maximum 5mg bd.

By mouth for restlessness and confusion

- *Child 1 month to 12 years*: initial dose of 50 micrograms/kg/24h (initial maximum 3mg/24h) in divided doses. The dose may be increased, as necessary, to a maximum of 170 micrograms/kg/24h in divided doses.
- *Child 12–18 years*: 10–20 micrograms/kg every 8–12h; maximum 10mg/day.

By mouth for intractable hiccups

- *Child 1 month to 12 years*: initial dose of 50 micrograms/kg/24h (initial maximum 3mg/24h) in divided doses. The dose may be increased, as necessary, to a maximum of 170 micrograms/kg/24h in divided doses.
- *Child 12–18 years*: 1.5mg tds.

By continuous intravenous or subcutaneous infusion (for any indication)

- *Child 1 month to 12 years*: initial dose of 25 micrograms/kg/24h (initial maximum 1.5mg/24h). The dose may be increased, as necessary, to a maximum of 85 micrograms/kg/24h.
- *Child 12–18 years*: initial dose of 1.5mg/24h. The dose may be increased, as necessary, to a suggested maximum of 5mg/24h, although higher doses may be used under specialist advice.

Notes

- D_2 receptor antagonist and typical antipsychotic.
- Not licensed for use in children with nausea and vomiting, restlessness and confusion, or intractable hiccups. Injection is licensed only for im administration in adults; iv and sc administration off-label (all ages).
- Haloperidol can cause potentially fatal prolongation of the QT interval and torsades de pointes, particularly if given iv (off-label route) or at higher than recommended doses. Caution is required if any formulation of haloperidol is given to patients with an underlying predisposition, e.g. those with cardiac abnormalities, hypothyroidism, familial long QT syndrome, electrolyte imbalance, or taking other drugs known to prolong the QT interval. If iv haloperidol is essential, ECG monitoring during drug administration is recommended.

- Dosages for restlessness and confusion are often higher.
- Adult dosages can exceed 15mg/24h in severe agitation.
- Oral doses are based on an oral bioavailability of ~50% of the parenteral route, i.e. oral doses ~2× parenteral.
- Useful as long-acting—od dosing is often adequate.
- Oral solutions may be administered via an enteral feeding tube.
- Available as: tablets (500 micrograms, 1.5mg, 5mg, 10mg, 20mg), capsules (500 micrograms), oral liquid (1mg/mL, 2mg/mL), and injection (5mg/mL).

Hydromorphone

Uses
- Alternative opioid analgesic for severe pain, especially if intolerant to other strong opioids.
- Antitussive.

Dose and routes
Normally convert using OME from previous analgesia.

Use the following *starting* doses in opioid-naïve patient. The maximum dose stated applies to the *starting* dose only.

By mouth
- *Child 1–18 years*: 30 micrograms/kg per dose; maximum 2mg per dose every 3–4h, increasing as required. Modified-release capsules with an initial dose of 4mg every 12h may be used from 12 years of age.

By intravenous or subcutaneous injection
- *Child 1–18 years*: initially 15 micrograms/kg per dose slowly over at least 2–3min every 3–6h.
- Convert from oral (halve the dose for equivalence).

Notes
- Hydrated morphine ketone effects are common to the class of mu agonist analgesics.
- Injection is not licensed in the UK. May be possible to obtain via a specialist importation company, but as hydromorphone is a CD, this is not a straightforward process.
- Oral form licensed for use in children from 12 years of age with cancer pain.
- Oral bioavailability 37–62% (wide inter-individual variation), onset of action 15min for sc, 30min for po. Peak plasma concentration 1h po. Plasma half-life 2.5h early phase, with a prolonged late phase. Duration of action 4–5h.
- Potency ratios seem to vary more than for other opioids. This may be due to inter-individual variation in metabolism or bioavailability.
- Conversion of po morphine to po hydromorphone: divide the morphine dose by 5–7.

- Conversion of iv morphine to iv hydromorphone: divide the morphine dose by 5–7.
- Dosage discontinuation: after short-term therapy (7–14 days), the original dose can be decreased by 10–20% of the original dose every 8h, increasing gradually the time interval. After long-term therapy, the dose should be reduced not more than 10–20% per week.
- Caution in hepatic impairment; use at reduced starting doses.
- Modified-release capsules are given 12-hourly.
- Capsules (both types) can be opened, and contents sprinkled on soft food. Capsule contents must not, however, be administered via an enteral feeding tube, as likely to cause blockage.
- Available as: capsules (1.3mg, 2.6mg) and modified-release capsules (2mg, 4mg, 8mg, 16mg, 24mg).

Hyoscine butylbromide

Uses
- Adjuvant where pain is caused by spasm of the gastrointestinal or genitourinary tract.
- Management of secretions, especially where drug crossing the blood–brain barrier is an issue.

Dose and routes
By mouth or intramuscular or intravenous injection
- *Child 1 month to 4 years*: 300–500 micrograms/kg (maximum 5mg/dose) 3–4 times daily.
- *Child 5–12 years*: 5–10mg 3–4 times daily.
- *Child 12–18 years*: 10–20mg 3–4 times daily.

By continuous subcutaneous infusion
- *Child 1 month to 4 years*: 1.5mg/kg/24h (maximum 15mg/24h).
- *Child 5–12 years*: 30mg/24h.
- *Child 12–18 years*: up to 60–80mg/24h.
- Higher doses may be needed; doses used in adults range from 20 to 120mg/24h (maximum dose 300mg/24h).

Notes
- Does not cross the blood–brain barrier (unlike hyoscine hydrobromide), hence no central antiemetic effect and does not cause drowsiness.
- Tablets are not licensed for use in children <6 years old.
- Injection is not licensed for use in children.
- The injection solution may be given po or via an enteral feeding tube. If the tube exits in the jejunum, consider using parenteral therapy. Injection solution can be stored for 24h in the refrigerator.
- iv injection should be given slowly over 1min and can be diluted with 5% glucose or 0.9% NaCl.
- Available as: tablets (10mg) and injection (20mg/mL).

Hyoscine hydrobromide

Uses
- Control of upper airways secretions and hypersalivation.

Dose and routes
By mouth or sublingual
- *Child 2–12 years*: 10 micrograms/kg (maximum 300 micrograms single dose) qds.
- *Child 12–18 years*: 300 micrograms qds.

By transdermal route
- *Child 1 month to 3 years*: quarter of a patch every 72h.
- *Child 3–10 years*: half of a patch every 72h.
- *Child 10–18 years*: one patch every 72h.

By subcutaneous or intravenous injection or infusion
- *Child 1 month to 18 years*: 10 micrograms/kg (maximum 600 micrograms) every 4–8h or CSCI/iv infusion 40–60 micrograms/kg/24h. Maximum suggested dose is 2.4mg in 24h, although higher doses are often used by specialist units.

Notes
- Not licensed for use in children for control of upper airways secretion and hypersalivation.
- Higher doses often used under specialist advice.
- Can cause delirium or sedation (sometimes paradoxical stimulation) with repeated dosing. Constipating.
- Apply the patch to a hairless area of skin behind the ear.
- The patch can cause alteration of the pupil size on the side it is placed.
- Some specialists advise that transdermal patches should not be cut—however, the manufacturers of Scopoderm TTS® patch have confirmed that it is safe to do this.
- Injection solution may be administered po.
- Available as: tablets (150 micrograms, 300 micrograms), patches (releasing 1mg/72h), and injection (400 micrograms/mL, 600 micrograms/mL). An oral solution is available via a 'specials' manufacturer.

Ibuprofen

Uses
- Simple analgesic.
- Pyrexia.
- Adjuvant for musculoskeletal pain.

Dose and routes
By mouth
- *Neonate*: 5mg/kg/dose every 12h.
- *Child 1–3 months*: 5mg/kg 3–4 times daily, preferably after food.

- *Child 3–6 months*: 50mg tds, preferably after food; in severe conditions, up to 30mg/kg daily in 3–4 divided doses.
- *Child 6 months to 1 year*: 50mg 3–4 times daily, preferably after food; in severe conditions, up to 30mg/kg daily in 3–4 divided doses.
- *Child 1–4 years*: 100mg tds, preferably after food. In severe conditions, up to 30mg/kg daily in 3–4 divided doses.
- *Child 4–7 years*: 150mg tds, preferably after food. In severe conditions, up to 30mg/kg daily in 3–4 divided doses.
- *Child 7–10 years*: 200mg tds, preferably after food. In severe conditions, up to 30mg/kg daily in 3–4 divided doses. Maximum daily dose 2.4g.
- *Child 10–12 years*: 300mg tds, preferably after food. In severe conditions, up to 30mg/kg daily in 3–4 divided doses. Maximum daily dose 2.4g.
- *Child 12–18 years*: 300–400mg 3–4 times daily, preferably after food. In severe conditions, the dose may be increased to a maximum of 2.4g/day.

Pain and inflammation in rheumatic diseases, including idiopathic juvenile arthritis
- *Child aged 3 months to 8 years and body weight >5kg*: 30–40mg/kg daily in 3–4 divided doses, preferably after food. Maximum 2.4g daily.

In systemic juvenile idiopathic arthritis
- Up to 60mg/kg daily in 4–6 divided doses, up to a maximum of 2.4g daily (off-label).

Notes
- Will cause closure of ductus arteriosus; contraindicated in duct-dependent congenital heart disease.
- Orphan drug licence for closure of ductus arteriosus in preterm neonate.
- Not licensed for use in children under 3 months of age or weight <5kg.
- Topical preparations and granules are not licensed for use in children.
- Ibuprofen combines anti-inflammatory, analgesic, and antipyretic properties. It has fewer side effects than other NSAIDs, but its anti-inflammatory properties are weaker.
- The risk of cardiovascular events secondary to NSAID use is undetermined in children. In adults, all NSAID use (including COX-2 selective inhibitors) can, to varying degrees, be associated with a small increased risk of thrombotic events (e.g. myocardial infarction and stroke), independent of baseline cardiovascular risk factors or duration of NSAID use; however, the greatest risk may be in those patients receiving high doses long-term. A small increased thrombotic risk cannot be excluded in children.
- All NSAIDs are associated with gastrointestinal toxicity. In adults, evidence on the relative safety of NSAIDs indicates differences in the risks of serious upper gastrointestinal side effects—piroxicam and ketorolac are associated with the highest risk; indometacin, diclofenac, and naproxen are associated with intermediate risk, and ibuprofen with the lowest risk (although high doses of ibuprofen have been associated with intermediate risk).

- Caution in asthma, and look out for symptoms and signs of gastritis.
- Consider the use of a PPI with prolonged use of ibuprofen.
- For administration via an enteral feeding tube, use a liquid preparation; dilute with an equal volume of water immediately prior to administration where possible.
- Available as: tablets (200mg, 400mg, 600mg), capsule (300mg modified-release), oral syrup (100mg/5mL), granules (600mg/sachet), and spray, creams, and gels (5%).

Ipratropium bromide

Uses

- Wheezing/breathlessness caused by bronchospasm.

Dose and routes

Nebulized solution

- *Child <1 year*: 62.5 micrograms 3–4 times daily.
- *Child 1–5 years*: 125–250 micrograms 3–4 times daily.
- *Child 5–12 years*: 250–500 micrograms 3–4 times daily.
- *Child over 12 years*: 500 micrograms 3–4 times daily.

Aerosol inhalation

- *Child 1 month to 6 years*: 20 micrograms tds.
- *Child 6–12 years*: 20–40 micrograms tds.
- *Child 12–18 years*: 20–40 micrograms 3–4 times daily.

Notes

- Inhaled product should be used with a suitable spacer device, and the child/carer should be given appropriate training.
- In acute asthma, use via an oxygen-driven nebulizer.
- In severe acute asthma, the dose can be repeated every 20–30min in the first 2h, then every 4–6h, as necessary.
- Available as: nebulizer solution (250 micrograms in 1mL, 500 micrograms in 2mL) and aerosol inhaler (20 micrograms per metered dose).

Ketamine

Uses

- Adjuvant to a strong opioid for neuropathic pain.
- To reduce NMDA receptor wind-up pain and opioid tolerance.

Dose and routes

By mouth or sublingual

- *Child 1 month to 12 years*: starting dose 150 micrograms/kg, as required or regularly 6- to 8-hourly; increase in increments of 150 micrograms/kg up to 400 micrograms/kg, as required. Doses equivalent to 3mg/kg have been reported in adults.

- *Over 12 years and adult*: 10mg, as required or regularly 6- to 8-hourly; increase in steps of 10mg up to 50mg, as required. Doses up to 200mg qds reported in adults.

By continuous subcutaneous or intravenous infusion
- *Child 1 month to adult*: starting dose 40 micrograms/kg/h. Increase according to response; usual maximum 100 micrograms/kg/h. Doses up to 1.5mg/kg/h in children and 2.5mg/kg/h in adults have been reported.

Notes
- NMDA antagonist.
- Specialist use only.
- Not licensed for use in children with neuropathic pain.
- Higher doses (bolus injection 1–2mg/kg, infusions 600–2700 micrograms/kg/h) used as an anaesthetic, e.g. for short procedures.
- Sublingual doses should be prepared in a maximum volume of 2mL. The bitter taste may make this route unpalatable. Special preparations for sublingual use are available in the UK.
- Enteral dose equivalents may be as low as one-third of iv or sc dose, because ketamine is potentiated by hepatic first-pass metabolism. Other papers quote a 1:1 sc to po conversion ratio.
- Agitation, hallucinations, anxiety, dysphoria, and sleep disturbance are recognized side effects. These may be less common in children and when sub-anaesthetic doses are used.
- Ketamine can cause urinary tract symptoms—frequency, urgency, dysuria, and haematuria. Consider discontinuing ketamine if these symptoms occur.
- Caution in severe hepatic impairment; consider dose reduction.
- Dilute in 0.9% saline for sc or iv infusion.
- Can be administered as a separate infusion or by adding to opioid infusion/PCA/nurse-controlled analgesia (NCA).
- Can also be used intranasally and as a topical gel.
- Available as: injection (10mg/mL, 50mg/mL, 100mg/mL) and oral solution 50mg in 5mL (from a 'specials' manufacturer). Injection solution may be given po. Mix with a flavoured soft drink to mask the bitter taste.

Ketorolac

Uses
- Short-term management of moderate to severe acute post-operative pain; limited evidence of extended use in chronic pain.

Dose and routes
Short-term management of moderate to severe acute post-operative pain (NB. licensed duration is a maximum of 2 days; not licensed for use in adolescents and children <16 years of age)
Intravenous bolus (over at least 15s) or intramuscular bolus
- *Child 1–16 years*: initially 0.5–1mg/kg (maximum 10mg), then 500 micrograms/kg (maximum 15mg) every 6h, as required; maximum 60mg daily.

- *Child >16 years*: initially 10mg, then 10–30mg every 4–6h, as required (up to every 2h during initial post-operative period); maximum 90mg daily (those weighing <50kg: maximum 60mg daily).

Chronic pain in palliative care (unlicensed indication; data limited and of poor quality; anecdotal reports of effectiveness for patients with bone pain unresponsive to oral NSAIDs)

Subcutaneous bolus
- *Child >16 years*: 15–30mg/dose tds.

Continuous subcutaneous infusion
- *Child >16 years*: initial dose of 60mg/24h. Increase, if necessary, by 15mg/24h to a maximum of 90mg/24h.

Notes
- NSAID which has potent analgesic effects, with only moderate anti-inflammatory action.
- Licensed only for the short-term management (maximum of 2 days) of moderate to severe acute post-operative pain in adults and adolescents from 16 years of age.
- sc administration is an unlicensed route of administration.
- Contraindications: previous hypersensitivity to ketorolac or other NSAIDs; history of asthma; active peptic ulcer or history of gastrointestinal bleeding; severe heart, hepatic, or renal failure; suspected or confirmed cerebrovascular bleeding or coagulation disorders. Do not use in combination with any other NSAID.
- Dose in adults with mild renal impairment should not exceed 60mg/day.
- All NSAIDs are associated with gastrointestinal toxicity. In adults, evidence on the relative safety of NSAIDs indicates ketorolac and piroxicam are associated with the highest risk. Use the lowest effective dose for the shortest time. In addition, consider use in combination with a gastroprotective drug, especially if ketorolac is used for a prolonged period (outside the licensed indication). Use of ketorolac in adults carries a 15 times increased risk of upper gastrointestinal complications, and a three times increased risk, compared with other non-selective NSAIDs.
- In adults, all NSAID use can, to varying degrees, be associated with a small increased risk of thrombotic effects. The risk of cardiovascular effects secondary to NSAID use is undetermined in children, but, in adults, ketorolac is associated with the highest myocardial infarction risk of all NSAIDs.
- Other potential adverse effects: very common (>10% of patients)—headache, dyspepsia, nausea, abdominal pain; common (1–10% of patients)—dizziness, tinnitus, oedema, hypertension, anaemia, stomatitis, abnormal renal function, pruritus, purpura, rash, bleeding, and pain at injection site. Risk of adverse effects likely to increase with prolonged use.
- Drug interactions include: anticoagulants (contraindicated, as the combination may cause an enhanced anticoagulant effect); corticosteroids (increased risk of gastrointestinal ulceration of

bleeding); diuretics (risk of reduced diuretic effect and increased risk of nephrotoxicity of NSAIDs); other potential nephrotoxic drugs.

- Onset of action iv/im injection: 10–30min; maximal analgesia achieved within 1–2h and median duration of effect 4–6h.
- sc injection can be irritant; therefore, dilute to the largest volume possible (0.9% NaCl suggested). Alkaline in solution, so high risk of incompatibility mixed with acidic drugs. Some data of compatibility in 0.9% saline with diamorphine or oxycodone. Incompatibilities include with cyclizine, glycopyrronium, haloperidol, levomepromazine, midazolam, and morphine.
- Available as: injection (30mg/mL). Injection contains ethanol as an excipient.
- Oral 10mg tablets and injection 10mg/mL no longer available in the UK (discontinued early 2013 due to lack of demand).

Lactulose

Uses

- Constipation, faecal incontinence related to constipation.
- Hepatic encephalopathy and coma.

Dose and routes

Constipation

By mouth: initial dose bd, then adjusted to suit the patient.

- *Neonate*: 2.5mL/dose bd.
- *Child 1 month to 1 year*: 2.5mL/dose 1–3 times daily.
- *Child 1–5 years*: 5mL/dose 1–3 times daily.
- *Child 5–10 years*: 10mL/dose 1–3 times daily.
- *Child 10–18 years*: 15mL/dose 1–3 times daily.

Hepatic encephalopathy

- *Child 12–18 years*: use 30–50mL tds as initial dose. Adjust dose to produce 2–3 soft stools per day.

Notes

- Licensed for constipation in all age groups. Not licensed for hepatic encephalopathy in children.
- Side effects may cause nausea and flatus, with colic especially at high doses. Initial flatulence usually settles after a few days.
- Precautions and contraindications: galactosaemia, intestinal obstruction. Caution in lactose intolerance.
- Use is limited, as macrogols are often better in palliative care. However, the volume per dose of macrogols is 5–10 times greater than lactulose and may not be tolerated in some patients.
- Sickly taste.
- Onset of action can take 36–48h.
- May be taken with water and other drinks.
- Relatively ineffective in opioid-induced constipation: need a stimulant.

- 15mL/day is 14kcal, so unlikely to affect diabetics.
- Does not irritate or directly interfere with gut mucosa.
- Available as: oral solution (10g/15mL). Cheaper than Movicol®
  (macrogol).

Lansoprazole

Uses
- GORD; erosive oesophagitis; prevention and treatment of NSAID
  gastric and oesophageal irritation; treatment of duodenal and
  gastric ulcer.

Dose and routes
Oral
- *Child body weight <30kg*: 0.5–1mg/kg with maximum 15mg od in the
  morning.
- *Child body weight >30kg*: 15–30mg od in the morning.

Notes
- Lansoprazole is not licensed in the UK for infants, children, or
  adolescents. Lansoprazole is, however, licensed in the USA for use from
  1 year of age. Exact doses limited by available formulations.
- Lansoprazole is a gastric PPI. It inhibits the final stage of gastric acid
  formation by inhibiting the activity of H^+/K^+ ATPase of the parietal cells
  in the stomach. The inhibition is dose-dependent and reversible, and the
  effect applies to both basal and stimulated secretion of gastric acid.
- For optimal effect, the single daily dose is best taken in the morning.
- Lansoprazole should be taken at least 30min before food, as intake with
  food slows down the absorption and decreases the bioavailability.
- The dose may be increased if symptoms do not fully resolve (consider
  increasing the single daily dose or bd dosing).
- Studies in infants and children indicate they appear to need a higher mg/
  kg dose than adults to achieve therapeutic acid suppression.
- There is some anecdotal experience that lansoprazole FasTab® may be
  halved to give a 7.5mg dose.
- No dose adjustment is needed in patients with renal impairment.
  Reduction of dose (50%) is recommended in patients with moderate to
  severe hepatic impairment.
- Hypomagnesaemia may develop with prolonged use.
- Common adverse effects (>1 in 100 to <1 in 10): headache, dizziness,
  nausea, diarrhoea, stomach pain, constipation, vomiting, flatulence, dry
  mouth, pharyngitis, increase in liver enzyme levels, urticaria, itching,
  and rash.
- Lansoprazole may interfere with absorption of drugs where gastric pH
  is critical to its bioavailability (e.g. atazanavir, itraconazole); may cause
  increase in digoxin levels and increase in plasma concentration of drugs
  metabolized by CYP3A4 (e.g. theophylline and tacrolimus). Drugs
  which inhibit or induce CYP2C19 or CYP3A4 may affect the plasma

concentration of lansoprazole. Sucralfate and antacids may decrease the bioavailability of lansoprazole.

- Capsules: capsules should be swallowed whole with liquid. For patients with difficulty swallowing, studies and clinical practice suggest that the capsules may be opened, and the granules mixed with a small amount of water or apple/tomato juice, or sprinkled onto a small amount of soft food (e.g. yoghurt, apple puree) to ease administration.
- FasTab®: place on the tongue, and gently suck. FasTab® rapidly disperses in the mouth, releasing gastro-resistant microgranules which are then swallowed. FasTab® can be swallowed whole with water or mixed with a small amount of water, if preferred. FasTab® contains lactose and aspartame and should be used with caution in known phenylketonuria (PKU) patients.
- For administration via an NG or gastrostomy tube, lansoprazole FasTab® can be dispersed in 10mL of water and administered via an 8Fr NG tube without blockage. For smaller-bore tubes, dissolve the contents of a lansoprazole capsule in 8.4% sodium bicarbonate before administration. If the tube becomes blocked, use sodium bicarbonate to dissolve any enteric-coated granules lodged in the tube. Lansoprazole less likely than omeprazole MUPS to cause blockage of small-bore tubes.
- Available as: 15mg and 30mg capsules, and 15mg and 30mg orodispersible tablets including FasTab® (Zoton®).

Levomepromazine

Uses

- Broad-spectrum antiemetic where the cause is unclear or where probably multifactorial.
- Second-line if a specific antiemetic fails.
- Severe pain unresponsive to other measures—may be of benefit in a very distressed patient.
- Sedation for terminal agitation, particularly in end-of-life care.

Dose and routes

Used as antiemetic

By mouth
- *Child 2–12 years*: initial dose 50–100 micrograms/kg, given od or bd. This dose may be increased, as necessary and as tolerated, not to exceed 1mg/kg/dose (or maximum of 25mg/dose), given od or bd.
- *Child 12–18 years*: initial dose 3mg od or bd. This dose may be increased, as necessary and as tolerated, to a maximum of 25mg od or bd.

By continuous intravenous or subcutaneous infusion over 24h
- *Child 1 month to 12 years*: initial dose of 100 micrograms/kg/24h, increasing, as necessary, to a maximum of 400 micrograms/kg/24h. Maximum 25mg/24h.
- *Child 12–18 years*: initial dose of 5mg/24h, increasing, as necessary, to a maximum of 25mg/24h.

Used for sedation

By subcutaneous infusion over 24h
- *Child 1–12 years*: initial dose of 350 micrograms/kg/24h (maximum initial dose 12.5mg), increasing, as necessary, up to 3mg/kg/24h.
- *Child 12–18 years*: initial dose of 12.5mg/24h, increasing, as necessary, up to 200mg/24h.

Analgesia
- In adults, stat dose 12.5mg/dose by mouth or sc. Titrate the dose according to response; usual maximum daily dose in adults is 100mg sc or 200mg by mouth.

Notes
- Licensed for use in children with terminal illness for the relief of pain and accompanying anxiety and distress.
- A low dose is often effective as antiemetic. Titrate up, as necessary. Higher doses are very sedative, and this may limit dose increases.
- If the child is not stable on high dosage for nausea and vomiting, reconsider the cause, and combine with other agents.
- Some experience in adults with low dose used buccally as antiemetic (e.g. 1.5mg tds as needed).
- Can cause hypotension, particularly with higher doses. Somnolence and asthenia are frequent side effects.
- Levomepromazine and its non-hydroxylated metabolites are reported to be potent inhibitors of cytochrome P450 2D6. Co-administration of levomepromazine and drugs primarily metabolized by the cytochrome P450 2D6 enzyme system may result in increased plasma concentrations of these drugs that could increase or prolong both their therapeutic and/or adverse effects.
- Avoid, or use with caution, in patients with liver dysfunction or cardiac disease.
- Tablets may be halved or quartered to obtain smaller doses. Tablets/segments may be dispersed in water for administration via an enteral feeding tube.
- For sc infusion, dilute with 0.9% NaCl. WFI may also be used. The sc dose is considered to be twice as potent as that administered po.
- Available as: tablets (25mg) and injection (25mg/mL). A 6mg tablet is also available via specialist importation companies. An extemporaneous oral solution may be prepared.

Lidocaine (lignocaine) patch

Uses
- Localized neuropathic pain.

Dose and routes
Topical
- *Child 3–18 years*: apply 1–2 plasters to affected area(s). Apply the plaster od for 12h, followed by a 12h plaster-free period (to help reduce the risk of skin reactions).
- *Adult 18 years or above*: up to three plasters to affected area(s). Apply the plaster od for 12h, followed by a 12h plaster-free period (to help reduce the risk of skin reactions).

Notes
- Not licensed for use in children or adolescents under 18 years.
- Cut the plaster to size and shape of the painful area. Do NOT use on broken or damaged skin or near the eyes.
- When lidocaine 5% medicated plaster is used according to the maximum recommended dose (three plasters applied simultaneously for 12h), about 3 ± 2% of the total applied lidocaine dose is systemically available, and similar for single and multiple administrations.
- Maximum recommended number of patches in adults currently is three per application.
- The plaster contains propylene glycol which may cause skin irritation. It also contains methyl parahydroxybenzoate and propyl parahydroxybenzoate which may cause allergic reactions (possibly delayed). ~16% of patients can be expected to experience adverse reactions. These are localized reactions due to the nature of the medicinal product.
- The plaster should be used with caution in patients with severe cardiac impairment, severe renal impairment, or severe hepatic impairment.
- A recent analysis by anatomic site of patch placement suggests that application to the head was tolerated less well, compared with the trunk and extremities.
- Doses extrapolated from *BNF* 2012 March.
- Available as: 700mg/medicated plaster (5% w/v lidocaine).

Lomotil® (co-phenotrope)

Uses
- Diarrhoea from non-infectious cause.

Dose and routes
By mouth
- *Child 2–4 years*: half tablet tds.
- *Child 4–9 years*: one tablet tds.
- *Child 9–12 years*: one tablet qds.

- *Child 12–16 years*: two tablets tds.
- *Child 16–18 years*: initially four tablets, then two tablets qds.

Notes

- Not licensed for use in children <4 years.
- Tablets may be crushed. For administration via an enteral feeding tube, tablets may be crushed and dispersed in water immediately before use. Young children are particularly susceptible to overdosage, and symptoms may be delayed, and observation is needed for at least 48h after ingestion. Overdose can be difficult to manage, with a mixed picture of opioid and atropine poisoning. Further, the presence of subclinical doses of atropine may give rise to atropine side effects in susceptible individuals.
- Available only as: tablets of co-phenotrope (2.5mg diphenoxylate hydrochloride and 25 micrograms atropine sulfate).

Loperamide

Uses

- Diarrhoea from non-infectious cause.
- Faecal incontinence.

Dose and routes

By mouth

- *Child 1 month to 1 year*: initial dose of 100 micrograms/kg bd, given 30min before feeds. Increase, as necessary, up to a maximum of 2mg/kg/day, given in divided doses.
- *Child 1–12 years*: initial dose of 100 micrograms/kg (maximum single dose 2mg) 3–4 times daily. Increase, as necessary, up to a maximum of 1.25mg/kg/day, given in divided doses (maximum 16mg/day).
- *Child 12–18 years*: initial dose of 2mg 2–4 times daily. Increase, as necessary, up to a maximum of 16mg/day, given in divided doses.

Notes

- Not licensed for use in children with chronic diarrhoea.
- Capsules not licensed for use in children <8 years.
- Syrup not licensed for use in children <4 years.
- Common side effects: constipation, nausea, flatulence.
- As an antidiarrhoeal, loperamide is about 50 times more potent than codeine. It is longer-acting; maximum therapeutic impact may not be seen for 16–24h.
- For NG or gastrostomy administration: use the liquid preparation, undiluted. Flush well after dosing. Alternatively, the tablets can be used without risk of blockage, although efficacy is unknown. Jejunal administration will not affect the therapeutic response to loperamide. However, owing to the potential osmotic effect of the liquid preparation, it may be appropriate to further dilute the dose with water immediately prior to administration.
- Available as: tablets (2mg), orodispersible tablets (2mg), and oral syrup (1mg/5mL).

Lorazepam

Uses

- Background anxiety.
- Agitation and distress.
- Adjuvant in cerebral irritation.
- Background management of dyspnoea.
- Muscle spasm.
- Status epilepticus.

Dose and routes for all indications, except status epilepticus

By mouth

- *Child <2 years*: 25 micrograms/kg 2–3 times daily.
- *Child 2–5 years*: 500 micrograms 2–3 times daily.
- *Child 6–10 years*: 750 micrograms tds.
- *Child 11–14 years*: 1mg tds.
- *Child 15–18 years*: 1–2mg tds.

Sublingual

- *Children of all ages*: 25 micrograms/kg as a single dose. Increase to 50 micrograms/kg (maximum 1mg/dose), if necessary.
- *Usual adult dose*: 500 micrograms—1mg as a single dose; repeat as required.

Notes

- Not licensed for use in children for these indications other than status epilepticus.
- Tablets licensed in children over 5 years for premedication; injection not licensed in children <12 years, except for treatment of status epilepticus.
- Potency in the order of ten times that of diazepam per mg as anxiolytic/sedative.
- Well absorbed sublingually, with rapid onset of effect. There may, however, be variable absorption by this route, with further variation possible, depending on the formulation used; fast effect.
- Specific sublingual tablets are not available in the UK, but generic lorazepam tablets (specifically Genus, PVL, or TEVA brands) do dissolve in the mouth to be given sublingually.
- Tablets may be dispersed in water for administration via an enteral feeding tube.
- May cause drowsiness and respiratory depression, if given in large doses.
- Caution in renal and hepatic failure.
- Available as: tablets (1mg, 2.5mg) and injection (4mg in 1mL).

Macrogols: Movicol®

Uses
- Constipation.
- Faecal impaction.
- Suitable for opioid-induced constipation.

Dose and routes (Movicol® Paediatric for those <12 years of age; Movicol® from 12 years of age)
By mouth for constipation or prevention of faecal impaction
- *Child under 1 year*: half to one sachet daily.
- *Child 1–6 years*: one sachet daily (adjust dose according to response; maximum four sachets daily).
- *Child 6–12 years*: two sachets daily (adjust dose according to response; maximum four sachets daily).
- *Child 12–18 years*: 1–3 sachets daily of *adult* Movicol®.

By mouth for faecal impaction
- *Child under 1 year*: half to one sachet daily.
- *Child 1–5 years*: two sachets on the first day, and increase by two sachets every 2 days (maximum eight sachets daily). Treat until impaction resolved, then switch to maintenance laxative therapy.
- *Child 5–12 years*: four sachets on the first day, and increase by two sachets every 2 days (maximum 12 sachets daily). Treat until impaction resolved, then switch to maintenance laxative therapy.
- *Child 12–18 years*: four sachets daily of adult Movicol®, then increase by two sachets daily to a maximum of eight adult Movicol® sachets daily. Total daily dose should be drunk within a 6h period. After disimpaction, switch to maintenance laxative therapy.

Notes
- Not licensed for use in children <5 years with faecal impaction and <2 years with chronic constipation.
- Need to maintain hydration. Caution if fluid or electrolyte disturbance.
- Caution with high doses in those with impaired gag reflex, reflux oesophagitis, or impaired consciousness.
- Mix powder with water: Movicol® Paediatric 60mL per sachet and adult Movicol® 125mL per sachet.
- For administration via a feeding tube: dissolve the powder in water, as directed, and flush down the feeding tube. Flush well after dosing.
- Macrogol oral powder is also available as alternative brands Laxido Orange® and Molaxole®, but these preparations are licensed for use only from 12 years of age.

Melatonin

Uses
- Sleep disturbance due to disruption of circadian rhythm (*not* anxiolytic).

Dose and routes
By mouth
- *Child 1 month to 18 years*: initial dose 2–3mg, increasing every 1–2 weeks, dependent on effectiveness, up to maximum 12mg daily.

Notes
- Not licensed for use in children.
- Specialist use only.
- Some prescribers use a combination of immediate-release and modified-release tablets to optimize sleep patterns.
- Immediate-release capsules may be opened, and the contents sprinkled on cold food, if preferred. Sustained-release capsules may also be opened, but the contents should not be chewed.
- Only licensed formulation in the UK is 2mg modified-release tablets. Various unlicensed formulations, including an immediate-release preparation, are available from 'specials' manufacturers or specialist importing companies.

Methadone

(WARNING: requires additional training for dosing.)

Uses
- Major opioid used for moderate to severe pain, particularly neuropathic pain and pain poorly responsive to other opioids.
- Not normally used as first-line analgesia.

Caution
- Methadone should only be commenced by practitioners experienced in its use.
- This is due to wide inter-individual variation in response, very variable conversion ratios with other opioids, complex pharmacokinetics, and a long half-life.
- Initial close monitoring is particularly important.

Dose and routes
In opioid-naïve children

By mouth, and subcutaneous and intravenous injection
- *Child 1–12 years*: 100–200 micrograms/kg every 4h for first 2–3 doses, then every 6–12h (maximum dose 5mg/dose initially).
- Methadone has a long and variable half-life, with potential to cause sedation, respiratory depression, and even death from secondary peak phenomenon.

- Titration of methadone dosing must be done under close clinical observation of the patient, particularly in the first few days. Due to a large volume of distribution, higher doses are required for the first few days, while body tissues become saturated. Once saturation is complete, a smaller dose is sufficient. Continuing on the initial daily dose is likely to result in sedation within a few days, possible respiratory depression, and even death.
- *Doses may need to be reduced by up to 50% 2–3 days after the initial effective dose has been found to prevent adverse effects*, due to tissue saturation and methadone accumulation. From then on, increments in methadone dosing should be approximately at weekly intervals, with a maximum increase of 50% (experienced practitioners may increase more frequently).
- Continued clinical reassessment is required to avoid toxicity, as the time to reach steady-state concentration, following a change in dosing, may be up to 12 days.
- For breakthrough pain, we would recommend using a short half-life opioid.

In opioid substitution/rotation or switch
Caution
Substitution, rotation, or switch to methadone is a specialist skill and should only be undertaken in close collaboration with practitioners experienced in its use. There is a risk of unexpected death through overdose.

Equianalgesic doses

Dose conversion ratios from other opioids are not static but are a function of previous opioid exposure and are highly variable.

Published tables of equianalgesic doses of opioids, established in healthy, non-opioid-tolerant individuals, indicate that methadone is 1–2 times as potent as morphine in single dose studies, but, in individuals on long-term (and high-dose) morphine, methadone is closer to ten times as potent as morphine; it can be 30 times more potent or occasionally even more. The potency ratio tends to increase, as the dose of morphine increases. If considering methadone, thought should be given to the potential difficulty of subsequently switching from methadone to another opioid.

Other opioids should be considered first if switching from morphine, due to unacceptable effects or inadequate analgesia.

Consultation with a pain clinic or specialist palliative care service is advised.

In adults, there are several protocols for opioid rotation to methadone which are not evidence-based in paediatrics.

- In one approach, previous opioid therapy is completely stopped, before starting a fixed dose of methadone at variable dose intervals.
- The other approach incorporates a transition period where the dose of the former opioid is reduced and partially replaced by methadone which is then titrated upwards.

It can be difficult to convert a short-half-life opioid to a methadone equivalent dose and vice versa. Current practice is usually to admit to a specialist inpatient unit for 5–6 days of regular treatment or titrate orally at home with close supervision.

Converting oral methadone to subcutaneous/intravenous or continuous subcutaneous infusion/continuous intravenous infusion methadone

- Approximate dose ratios for switching between oral dosage and parenteral/sc form is 2:1 (oral:parenteral).
- Calculate the total daily dose of po methadone, and halve it (50%). This will be the 24h parenteral/sc methadone dose.
- Seek specialist guidance if mixing with any other drug.
- If CSCI methadone causes a skin reaction, consider doubling the dilution and changing the syringe every 12h.
- Administer iv methadone slowly over 3–5min.

Notes

- Not licensed for use in children.
- Data on methadone in paediatric patients are limited; known to have wide inter-individual pharmacokinetic variation.
- Use methadone with caution, as methadone's effect on respiration lasts longer than analgesic effects.
- Side effects include: nausea, vomiting, constipation, dry mouth, biliary spasm, respiratory depression, drowsiness, muscle rigidity, hypotension, bradycardia, tachycardia, palpitation, oedema, postural hypotension, hallucinations, vertigo, euphoria, dysphoria, dependence, confusion, urinary retention, ureteric spasm, and hypothermia.
- Following concerns regarding methadone and sudden death from prolongation of the QT interval or torsades de pointes (especially at high doses), it is recommended that patients have an ECG prior to initiation of treatment and regularly while on methadone, particularly if they have any risk factors or are having iv treatment of methadone.
- Opioid antagonists naloxone and naltrexone will precipitate an acute withdrawal syndrome in methadone-dependent individuals. Naloxone will also antagonize the analgesic, CNS, and respiratory depressant effects of methadone.
- Methadone has the potential for a number of significant drug interactions. Drugs that induce cytochrome P450 3A4 enzymes (e.g. carbamazepine, phenobarbital, phenytoin, rifampicin, some HIV drugs) will increase the rate of metabolism of methadone and potentially lead to reduced serum levels. Drugs that inhibit the system (e.g. amitriptyline, ciprofloxacin, fluconazole) may lead to increased serum levels of methadone.
- Renal impairment: if severe (i.e. glomerular filtration rate (GFR) <10mL/min or serum creatinine >700 micromoles/L)—reduce methadone dose by 50%, and titrate according to response. Significant accumulation is not likely in renal failure, as elimination is primarily via the liver.

- As methadone has a long half-life, infusion of naloxone may be required to treat opioid overdose.
- Available as: linctus (2mg/5mL), mixture (1mg/mL), solution (1mg/mL, 5mg/mL, 10mg/mL, and 20mg/mL), tablets (5mg), and injection (10mg/mL).

Methylnaltrexone

Uses

- Opioid-induced constipation when the response to other laxatives alone is inadequate and other relevant factors have been/are being addressed.

Dose and routes

Subcutaneous (usual route) or intravenous bolus

- *Child 1 month to 12 years*: 0.15mg/kg (maximum 8mg) as a single dose.
- *Child >12 years, with weight 38–61kg*: 8mg as a single dose.
- *Child >12 years, with weight 62–114kg*: 12mg as a single dose.
- *Child >12 years, but with body weight <38kg*: use 0.15mg/kg.

A single dose may be sufficient. However, repeat doses may be given, with a usual administration schedule of a single dose every other day. Doses may be given with longer intervals, as per clinical need. Patients may receive two consecutive doses (24h apart) only when there has been no response (no bowel movement) to the dose on the preceding day (one-third to half of patients given methylnaltrexone have a bowel movement within 4h, without loss of analgesia).

Notes

- Mu opioid receptor antagonist that acts exclusively in the peripheral tissues, including the gastrointestinal tract (increasing bowel movement and gastric emptying), and does not affect the analgesic effects of opioids.
- Not licensed for use in children or adolescents <18 years.
- Not licensed for iv administration—usual route is sc.
- Methylnaltrexone is contraindicated in cases of known or suspected bowel obstruction.
- The onset of effect may be within 15–60min.
- Common side effects include abdominal pain/colic, diarrhoea, flatulence, and nausea.
- If administered by sc injection, rotate the site of injection. Do not inject into areas where the skin is tender, bruised, red, or hard.
- Constipation in palliative care is usually multifactorial, and other laxatives are often required in addition.
- Reduce dose by 50% in severe renal impairment.
- Does not cross the blood–brain barrier.
- Available as: single-use vial 12mg/0.6mL solution for sc injection (Relistor®).

Metoclopramide

To minimize the risk of neurological side effects associated with metoclopramide, the EMA in 2013 issued the following recommendations *(NB. use of metoclopramide in palliative care was excluded from these recommendations. HOWEVER, caution should be exercised nevertheless)*:

- use of metoclopramide is contraindicated in children younger than 1 year;
- in children aged 1–18 years, metoclopramide should only be used as a second-line option for the prevention of delayed chemotherapy-induced nausea and vomiting (CINV) and for treatment of established post-operative nausea and vomiting (PONV);
- metoclopramide should only be prescribed for short-term use (up to 5 days).

Uses

- Antiemetic if vomiting caused by gastric compression or hepatic disease.
- Prokinetic for slow transit time (not in complete obstruction or with anticholinergics).
- Hiccups.

Dose and routes

By mouth, intramuscular injection, or intravenous injection (over at least 3min)

- *Neonate*: 100 micrograms/kg every 6–8h (by mouth or iv only).
- *Child 1 month to 1 year, with body weight up to 10kg*: 100 micrograms/kg (maximum 1mg/dose) bd.
- *Child 1–18 years*: 100–150 micrograms/kg, repeated up to tds. The maximum dose in 24h is 500 micrograms/kg (maximum 10mg/dose).

If preferred, the appropriate total daily dose may be administered as a continuous sc or iv infusion over 24h.

Notes

- Not licensed for use in infants <1 year of age.
- Not licensed for continuous iv or sc infusion.
- Metoclopramide can induce acute dystonic reactions such as facial and skeletal muscle spasms and oculogyric crises; children (especially girls, young women, and those under 10kg) are particularly susceptible. With metoclopramide, dystonic effects usually occur shortly after starting treatment and subside within 24h of stopping it.
- iv doses should be administered as a slow bolus over at least 3min to reduce the risk of adverse effects.
- Oral liquid formulations should be given via a graduated oral syringe to ensure dose accuracy in children. The oral liquid may be administered via an enteral feeding tube.
- Can be irritant on sc administration; dilute well in 0.9% NaCl.
- Available as: tablets (10mg), oral solution (5mg/5mL), and injection (5mg/mL).

Metronidazole topically

Uses
- Odour associated with fungating wounds or lesions.

Dose and routes
By topical application
- Apply to clean wound 1–2 times daily, and cover with non-adherent dressing.
- Cavities: smear gel on paraffin gauze, and pack loosely.

Notes
- Anabact® not licensed for use in children <12 years.
- Metrogel® not licensed for use in children.
- Available as: gel (Anabact® 0.75%, Metrogel® 0.75%).

Miconazole oral gel

Uses
- Oral and intestinal fungal infection.

Dose and routes
By mouth

Prevention and treatment of oral candidiasis
- *Neonate*: 1mL 2–4 times a day, smeared around the inside of the mouth after feeds.
- *Child 1 month to 2 years*: 1.25mL qds, smeared around the inside of the mouth after food.
- *Child 2–18 years*: 2.5mL qds after meals; retain near lesions before swallowing (orthodontic appliances should be removed at night and brushed with gel).

Prevention and treatment of intestinal candidiasis
- *Child 4 months to 18 years*: 5mg/kg qds; maximum 250mg (10mL) qds.

Notes
- Use after food, and retain near lesions before swallowing.
- Treatment should be continued for 7 days after lesions have healed.
- Not licensed for use in children under 4 months or during the first 5–6 months of life of an infant born preterm.
- Infants and babies: the gel should not be applied to the back of the throat, due to possible choking. The gel should not be swallowed immediately, but kept in the mouth for as long as possible.
- Available as: oral gel (24mg/mL in 15g and 80g tube).
- A buccal tablet of miconazole is now available. Indicated for the treatment of oropharyngeal candidiasis in immunocompromised adults. Loramyc® 50mg muco-adhesive buccal tablets should be applied to the upper gum, just above the incisor tooth, od for 7–14 days. Currently, no experience in children but may be an option for adolescents.

Midazolam

Uses

- Status epilepticus and terminal seizure control.
- Breakthrough anxiety, e.g. panic attacks.
- Adjuvant for pain of cerebral irritation.
- Anxiety-induced dyspnoea.
- Agitation at end of life.

Dose and routes

By oral or gastrostomy administration for anxiety or sedation
- *Child 1 month to 18 years*: 500 micrograms/kg (maximum 20mg) as a single dose.

Buccal doses for acute anxiety
- *Any age*: 100 micrograms/kg as a single dose (maximum initial dose 5mg).

By subcutaneous or intravenous infusion over 24h for anxiety
- Dosages of 30–50% of terminal seizure control dose can be used to control anxiety, terminal agitation, and terminal breathlessness.

Buccal doses for status epilepticus
- *Neonate*: 300 micrograms/kg as a single dose, repeated once if necessary.
- *Child 1–3 months*: 300 micrograms/kg (maximum initial dose 2.5mg), repeated once if necessary.
- *Child 3 months to 1 year*: 2.5mg, repeated once if necessary.
- *Child 1–5 years*: 5mg, repeated once if necessary.
- *Child 5–10 years*: 7.5mg, repeated once if necessary.
- *Child 10–18 years*: 10mg, repeated once if necessary.

By buccal or intranasal administration for *status epilepticus*—should wait 10min before repeating dose.

NB. In single dose for seizures, midazolam is twice as potent as pr diazepam. For patients who usually receive pr diazepam for the management of status epilepticus, consider an initial dose of buccal midazolam that is 50% of their usual pr diazepam dose to minimize the risk of respiratory depression.

By subcutaneous or intravenous infusion over 24h for terminal seizure control
- *Neonate (seizure control)*: 150 micrograms/kg iv loading dose, followed by a continuous iv infusion of 60 micrograms/kg/h. Dose can be increased by 60 micrograms/kg/h every 15min until seizure controlled (maximum dose 300 micrograms/kg/h).
- *Child 1 month to 18 years*: initial dose 50 micrograms/kg/h, increasing up to 300 micrograms/kg/h (maximum 100mg/24h or 150mg/24h in specialist units).

Notes

- Buccal (Buccolam® oromucosal solution) midazolam is not licensed for use in infants <3 months of age. Midazolam injection is not licensed for use in seizure control or anxiety.
- In single dose for sedation, midazolam is three times as potent as diazepam, and, in epilepsy, it is twice as potent as diazepam. (Diazepam gains in potency with repeated dosing because of prolonged half-life.)
- Recommended sc/iv doses vary enormously in the literature. If in doubt, start at the lowest recommended dose, and titrate rapidly.
- Onset of action by buccal and intranasal route 5–15min. For buccal administration, if possible, divide the dose, so half is given into one cheek, and the remaining half into the other cheek.
- Onset of action by po or gastrostomy route 10–30min.
- Onset of action by iv route 2–3min; sc route 5–10min.
- Midazolam has a short half-life.
- High doses can lead to paradoxical agitation.
- Available as: oral solution (2.5mg/mL unlicensed), buccal liquid (5mg/mL Buccolam®), and injection (1mg/mL, 2mg/mL, 5mg/mL).
- Other oral and buccal liquids (e.g. Epistatus® 10mg/mL) are also available from 'specials' manufacturers or specialist importing companies (unlicensed). NB. The buccal and oral formulations available may differ in strength—take care with prescribing.

Morphine

Uses

- Major opioid (WHO step 2).
- First-line oral opioid for pain.
- Dyspnoea.
- Cough suppressant.

Dose and routes

- Opioid-naïve patient: use the following start doses (the maximum dose stated applies to the *starting* dose only).
- Opioid conversion: convert using OME from the previous opioid.

By mouth or rectum

- *Child 1–3 months*: initially 50 micrograms/kg every 4h, adjusted according to response.
- *Child 3–6 months*: 100 micrograms/kg every 4h, adjusted according to response.
- *Child 6–12 months*: 200 micrograms/kg every 4h, adjusted according to response.
- *Child 1–12 years*: initially 200–300 micrograms/kg (initial maximum 5–10mg) every 4h, adjusted according to response.
- *Child 12–18 years*: initially 5–10mg every 4h, adjusted according to response.

By single subcutaneous injection or intravenous injection (over at least 5min)
- *Neonate*: initially 25 micrograms/kg every 6h, adjusted to response.
- *Child 1–6 months*: initially 50–100 micrograms/kg every 6h, adjusted to response.
- *Child 6 months to 2 years*: initially 100 micrograms/kg every 4h, adjusted to response.
- *Child 2–12 years*: initially 100 micrograms/kg every 4h, adjusted to response; maximum initial dose of 2.5mg.
- *Child 12–18 years*: initially 2.5–5mg every 4h, adjusted to response (maximum initial dose of 20mg/24h).

By continuous subcutaneous or intravenous infusion
- *Neonate*: 5 micrograms/kg/h, adjusted according to response.
- *Child 1–6 months*: 10 micrograms/kg/h, adjusted according to response.
- *Child 6 months to 18 years*: 20 micrograms/kg/h (maximum initial dose of 20mg/24h), adjusted according to response.

Parenteral dose: 30–50% of oral dose if converting from oral dose of morphine.

Dyspnoea
- 30–50% of the dose used for pain.

Notes
- *Oramorph®* solution not licensed for use in children under 1 year; *Oramorph®* unit dose vials not licensed for use in children under 6 years; *Sevredol®* tablets not licensed for use in children under 3 years; *Filnarine®* SR tablets not licensed for use in children under 6 years; *MST Continus®* preparations licensed to treat children with cancer pain (age range not specified by manufacturer); *MXL®* capsules not licensed for use in children under 1 year; suppositories not licensed for use in children. Caution in renal or hepatic impairment.
- Where opioid substitution or rotation is to morphine: use OME.
- Particular side effects include urinary retention and pruritus in the paediatric setting, in addition to well-recognized constipation, nausea, and vomiting.
- Morphine toxicity often presents as myoclonic twitching.
- Rectal route should be avoided, if possible, and is usually contraindicated in children with low platelets and/or neutropenia.
- In an emergency, when oral intake not appropriate, MST® tablets can be administered pr.
- Administration via enteral feeding tubes: for immediate pain relief, use oral solution; no further dilution is necessary. The tube must be flushed well, following dosing, to ensure that the total dose is delivered. For sustained pain relief, use MST Continus® sachets, dispersed in at least

10mL of water. Flush the tube well, following dosing, to ensure that the total dose is delivered. Note that any granules left in the tube will break down over a period of time, and a bolus of morphine will be delivered when the tube is next flushed; this has resulted in a reported fatality. Ensure that the dose prescribed can be administered using whole sachets when possible. Use of Zomorph® capsules opened to release the granules should be done with caution in children, due to issues with dose accuracy, and the granules should only be administered via an adult-size gastrostomy.

- Available as (all Schedule 2 CD, except oral solution of strength 10mg in 5mL):
  - tablets (10mg, 20mg, 50mg);
  - oral solution (10mg/5mL (POM), 100mg/5mL);
  - modified-release tablets and capsules 12-hourly (5mg, 10mg, 15mg, 30mg, 60mg, 100mg, 200mg);
  - modified-release suspension 12-hourly (20mg, 30mg, 60mg, 100mg, 200mg);
  - modified-release capsules 24-hourly (30mg, 60mg, 120mg, 150mg, 200mg);
  - suppositories (10mg, 15mg, 30mg);
  - injection (10mg/mL, 15mg/mL, 20mg/mL, 30mg/mL).

Nabilone

Uses

- Nausea and vomiting caused by cytotoxic chemotherapy (not first- or second-line therapy).
- For unresponsive nausea and vomiting to conventional antiemetics.

Dose and routes

By mouth

- *Adult dose*: 1–2mg bd (maximum dose 6mg/day in 2–3 divided doses).

Notes

- Not licensed for use in children.
- Nabilone is a synthetic cannabinoid.
- Individual variation, requiring close medical supervision on commencement and dose adjustments.
- The effects of nabilone may persist for a variable and unpredictable period of time, following its oral administration. Adverse psychiatric reactions can persist for 48–72h, following cessation of treatment.
- For specialist use only.
- Available as: capsules (1mg). Schedule 2 CD.

Naloxone

Uses
- Emergency use for reversal of opioid-induced respiratory depression or acute opioid overdose.
- Constipation when caused by opioids if methylnaltrexone not available and laxatives have been ineffective.

Dose and routes
Reversal of respiratory depression due to opioid overdose

By intravenous injection (review diagnosis; further doses may be required if respiratory depression deteriorates)
- *Neonate*: 10 micrograms/kg; if no response, give a subsequent dose of 100 micrograms/kg (then review diagnosis).
- *Child 1 month to 12 years*: 10 micrograms/kg; if no response, give a subsequent dose of 100 micrograms/kg (then review diagnosis).
- *Child 12–18 years*: 400 micrograms to 2mg; if no response, repeat at intervals of 2–3min to a maximum of 10mg total dose (then review diagnosis).

By subcutaneous or intramuscular injection only if intravenous route not feasible
- As per iv injection, but onset slower and potentially erratic.

By continuous intravenous infusion, adjusted according to response
- *Neonate*: rate adjusted to response (initially, rate may be set at 60% of the initial resuscitative iv injection dose per hour).
- *Child 1 month to 18 years*: rate adjusted to response (initially, rate may be set at 60% of the initial resuscitative iv injection dose per hour).
- *The initial resuscitative iv injection dose is that which maintained satisfactory self-ventilation for at least 15min.*

Opioid-induced constipation
By mouth
- In adults, the following doses have been used: total daily dose po naloxone = 20% of morphine dose; titrate according to need; maximum single dose 5mg.

Notes
- Potent opioid antagonist.
- Not licensed for use in children with constipation.
- Also see methylnaltrexone.
- Naloxone acts within 2min of iv injection and within 3–5min of sc or im injection.
- Although oral availability of naloxone is relatively low, be alert for opioid withdrawal symptoms, including recurrence of pain, at higher doses.
- Available as: injection (20 micrograms/mL, 400 micrograms/mL, 1mg/mL).

Naproxen

Uses
- Non-steroidal anti-inflammatory agent analgesic; relief of symptoms in inflammatory arthritis and treatment of acute musculoskeletal syndromes.

Dose and routes
- *Child 1 month to 18 years*: 5mg/kg/dose bd (maximum 1g/day).

Doses up to 10mg/kg bd (not exceeding 1g daily) have been used in severe conditions. High doses should ideally be used only for a short period. In general, use the lowest effective dose for the shortest treatment duration possible.

Notes
- Naproxen is licensed for use from 5 years of age for juvenile idiopathic arthritis; not licensed for use in children <16 years for other conditions.
- Naproxen is contraindicated in patients with a history of hypersensitivity to any NSAID or in those with a coagulation disorder.
- Use with caution in renal, cardiac, or hepatic failure, as this may cause a deterioration in renal function; the dose should be kept as low as possible, and renal function monitored. Avoid use if GFR <20mL/min/1.73m^2 and in those with severe hepatic or heart failure.
- Generally, naproxen is regarded as combining good efficacy with a low incidence of side effects.
- The risk of cardiovascular events secondary to NSAID use is undetermined in children. In adults, COX-2 selective inhibitors, diclofenac (150mg daily), and ibuprofen (2.4g daily) are associated with an increased risk of thrombotic effects (e.g. myocardial infarction and stroke). Naproxen (in adults 1g daily) is associated with a lower thrombotic risk. The greatest risk may increase with dose and duration of exposure, so the lowest effective dose should be used for the shortest possible duration of time.
- All NSAIDs are associated with gastrointestinal toxicity. In adults, evidence on the relative safety of NSAIDs indicates differences in the risks of serious upper gastrointestinal side effects—piroxicam and ketorolac are associated with the highest risk; indometacin, diclofenac, and naproxen are associated with intermediate risk, and ibuprofen with the lowest risk. Children appear to tolerate NSAIDs better than adults, and gastrointestinal side effects are less common, although they do still occur and can be significant.
- Other potential side effects include headache, dizziness, vertigo, fluid retention, and hypersensitivity reactions.
- The antipyretic and anti-inflammatory actions of naproxen may reduce fever and inflammation, therefore reducing their utility as diagnostic signs.
- Potential drug interactions include warfarin (increase in INR); and diuretics, ACE inhibitors, and angiotensin II antagonists (increased risk of compromised renal function). Naproxen is a substrate of CYP1A2

and CYP2C8/9 and can increase the plasma concentrations of
methotrexate and lithium.
- Naproxen tablets may be crushed before administration and can be mixed
with water for administration via a feeding tube. However, naproxen is
poorly soluble in water, and the tablet must be crushed to a fine powder
before mixing with water to avoid tube blockage. There may be better
choices of NSAID if administration via a feeding tube is necessary. Enteric-
coated naproxen tablets should be swallowed whole, and NOT be crushed
or chewed. Naproxen should be taken with or after food.
- Available as: tablets (250mg and 500mg), enteric-coated tablets (250mg
and 500mg), and oral suspension (25mg/mL, available only as a 'special'
from specials manufacturers).

Nystatin

Uses
- Oral and perioral fungal infection.

Dose and routes
By mouth
- *Neonate*: 100 000 units qds.
- *Child 1 month to 18 years*: 100 000 units qds.

Notes
- Licensed from 1 month of age for treatment. Neonates—nystatin is
licensed for prophylaxis against oral candidosis at a dose of 1mL daily.
- Retain near lesions before swallowing.
- Administer after food or feeds.
- Treatment for 7 days and should be continued for 48h after lesions have
healed.
- Available as: oral suspension (100 000 units/mL, 30mL with pipette).

Octreotide

Uses
- Bleeding from oesophageal or gastric varices.
- Nausea and vomiting.
- Intestinal obstruction.
- Intractable diarrhoea.
- Also used for hormone-secreting tumours, ascites, and bronchorrhoea.

Dose and routes
Bleeding from oesophageal varices

By continuous intravenous or subcutaneous infusion
- *Child 1 month to 18 years*: 1 microgram/kg/h. Higher doses may be
required initially. When there is no active bleeding, reduce dose over
24h. Usual maximum dose is 50 micrograms/h.

Nausea and vomiting, intestinal obstruction, and intractable diarrhoea
- By continuous iv or sc infusion: doses up to 1 microgram/kg/h have been used, but experience is limited. Do not stop abruptly—discontinue at a reducing rate.

Notes
- Not licensed for use in children.
- Administration: for iv injection or infusion, dilute with 0.9% NaCl to a concentration of 10–50% (i.e. not less than 1:1 and not more than 1:9 by volume). For sc bolus injections, may be administered neat, but this can be painful (this can be reduced if the ampoule is warmed in the hand to body temperature before injection). For sc infusion, dilute with 0.9% NaCl.
- Avoid abrupt withdrawal.
- Available as: injection for sc or iv administration (50 micrograms/mL, 100 micrograms/mL, 200 micrograms/mL, 500 micrograms/mL). Also available as depot injection for im administration every 28 days (10mg, 20mg, and 30mg Sandostatin Lar®). Recommend specialist palliative care advice.

Olanzapine

Uses
- Psychoses; delirium; agitation; nausea and vomiting; anorexia when all other treatments have failed.

Dose and routes
Oral

Psychoses/mania
- *Child <12 years and <25kg*: initial dose 2.5mg at night.
- *Child <12 years and >25kg*: initial dose 2.5–5mg at night.
- *Child 12–18 years*: initial dose 5mg at bedtime.

Increase gradually, as necessary and as tolerated, to a maximum of 20mg/day, given usually as a single dose at night.

Agitation/delirium
- *Child <12 years*: initial dose 1.25mg at night and prn.
- *Child 12–18 years*: initial dose 2.5mg at night and prn.

Increase gradually, as necessary and as tolerated, to maximum of 10mg/day.

Nausea and vomiting, and anorexia
- *Child <12 years*: initial dose 1.25mg (or 0.625mg if 2.5mg tablets can be cut into quarters) at night and prn.
- *Child 12–18 years*: initial dose 1.25–2.5mg at night and prn.

Dose may be increased, as necessary and as tolerated, to a suggested maximum of 7.5mg/day.

Notes

- Olanzapine is not licensed for use in children and adolescents <18 years of age, although there is general acknowledgement of 'off-label' use in adolescents for the treatment of psychosis and schizophrenia and mania associated with bipolar disorder.
- Use in the treatment of agitation/delirium, nausea and vomiting, and anorexia in palliative care are all 'off-label' indications.
- Olanzapine is an atypical (second-generation) antipsychotic agent and antagonist of D_1, D_2, D_3, D_4, $5HT_{2A}$, $5HT_3$, $5HT_6$, histamine-1, and muscarinic receptors.
- Olanzapine has five times the affinity for $5HT_2$ receptors than for D_2 receptors, resulting in fewer extrapyramidal side effects.
- Activity of olanzapine at multiple receptors is similar to methotrimeprazine, and therefore it has a potential role in the treatment of nausea and vomiting refractory to standard medication.
- Use with caution in those with cardiovascular disease or epilepsy (and conditions predisposing to seizures).
- Very common (>10% of patients) adverse effects: weight gain, elevated triglyceride levels, increased appetite, sedation, increased ALT and AST levels, decreased bilirubin, and increased gamma-glutamyl transpeptidase (GGT) and plasma prolactin levels. Common (1–10% of patients) adverse effects: elevated cholesterol levels, dry mouth.
- Rare, but potentially serious, adverse effects include neuroleptic malignant syndrome and neutropenia. Hyperglycaemia and sometime diabetes can occur.
- Dose titration should be slow to minimize sedation.
- A greater magnitude of weight gain and lipid and prolactin alterations have been reported in adolescents, compared to adults. If prolonged use is likely, consider the monitoring of blood lipids, weight, fasting blood glucose, and prolactin. Consider an ECG and BP measurement before initiation.
- Consider a lower starting dose (maximum 5mg in adults) in patients with renal and/or hepatic impairment.
- Olanzapine has good oral bioavailability, with peak plasma concentrations occurring within 5–8h. Absorption is not affected by food. Long elimination half-life of ~33h. Onset of actions is hours to days in delirium, and days to weeks in psychoses.
- Olanzapine does not inhibit or induce the main CYP450 isoenzymes. Olanzapine is metabolized by CYP1A2; therefore, drugs/substances that specifically induce or inhibit this isoenzyme may affect the pharmacokinetics of olanzapine, e.g. carbamazepine, fluvoxamine, nicotine.
- Orodispersible tablets: place in the mouth where the tablet will rapidly disperse in saliva or disperse in a full glass of water (or other drink) immediately before administration. May be dispersed in water for administration via an NG or gastrostomy feeding tube. Some anecdotal experience that 5mg orodispersible tablets may be halved to give a 2.5mg dose. Halve immediately before administration, and do not save the remaining half for a future dose.

- Coated tablets: swallow whole with liquid, or crushed and mixed with soft food.
- Orodispersible tablets contain aspartame and may be harmful for people with PKU.
- Coated tablets contain lactose.
- Available as: tablets (2.5mg, 5mg, 7.5mg, 10mg, 15mg, 20mg) and orodispersible tablets (5mg, 10mg, 15mg, 20mg).

Omeprazole

Uses
- Gastro-oesophageal reflux.
- Acid-related dyspepsia.
- Treatment of duodenal and gastric ulcers.
- Gastrointestinal prophylaxis (e.g. with combination NSAID/steroids).

Dose and routes
By mouth
- *Neonate*: 700 micrograms/kg od; increase, if necessary, to a maximum of 1.4mg/kg od (maximum dose 2.8mg/kg od).
- *Child 1 month to 2 years*: 700 micrograms/kg od; increase, if necessary, to a maximum of 3mg/kg od (maximum dose 20mg od).
- *Child body weight 10–20kg*: 10mg od; increase, if necessary, to a maximum of 20mg od.
- *Child body weight >20kg*: 20mg od; increase, if necessary, to a maximum of 40mg od.

Intravenous (by injection over 5min or by infusion over 20–30min)
- *Child 1 month to 12 years*: initially 500 micrograms/kg (maximum 20mg) od; increase, if necessary, to 2mg/kg (maximum 40mg) od.
- *Child 12–18 years*: 40mg od.

Notes
- Oral formulations are not licensed for use in children, except for severe ulcerating reflux oesophagitis in children >1 year.
- Injection not licensed for use in children under 12 years.
- Many children with life-limiting conditions have GORD and may need to continue with treatment long-term.
- Can cause agitation.
- Occasionally associated with electrolyte disturbance.
- For oral administration, tablets can be dispersed in water or with fruit juice or yoghurt. Capsules can be opened and mixed with fruit juice or yoghurt.
- Administer with care via enteral feeding tubes to minimize risk of blockage. Capsules may be opened, and contents dispersed in 8.4% sodium bicarbonate for administration. Dispersible tablets disintegrate to give a dispersion of small granules. The granules settle quickly and may block fine-bore feeding tubes (less than 8Fr).
- Available as: MUPS tablets (10mg, 20mg, 40mg), capsules (10mg, 20mg, 40mg), iv injection (40mg), iv infusion (40mg), and oral suspension available as special order (10mg/5mL).

Ondansetron

Uses

- Antiemetic, if vomiting caused by chemotherapy or radiotherapy.
- May have a use in managing opioid-induced pruritus.

Dose and routes

Prevention and treatment of chemotherapy- and radiotherapy-induced nausea and vomiting.

By intravenous infusion over at least 15min

- *Child 6 months to 18 years:* either 5mg/m^2 immediately before chemotherapy (maximum single dose 8mg), then give by mouth, *or* 150 micrograms/kg immediately before chemotherapy (maximum single dose 8mg), repeated every 4h for two further doses, then give by mouth; maximum total daily dose 32mg.

By mouth following intravenous administration

NB. Oral dosing can start 12h after iv administration.

- *Child 6 months to 18 years:*
  - body surface area <0.6m^2 *or* body weight 10kg or less: 2mg every 12h for up to 5 days (maximum total daily dose 32mg);
  - body surface area 0.6–1.2m^2 or greater *or* body weight over 10kg: 4mg every 12h for up to 5 days (maximum total daily dose 32mg);
  - body surface area >1.2m^2 *or* body weight over 40kg: 8mg every 12h for up to 5 days (maximum total daily dose 32mg).

Nausea and vomiting

By mouth or slow iv injection over 2–5min or by iv infusion over 15min.

- *Child 1–18 years:* 100–150 micrograms/kg/dose every 8–12h. Maximum single dose 4mg.

Notes

- Ondansetron injection is licensed for the management of CINV in children aged ≥6 months, and for the prevention and treatment of PONV in children (as a single dose) aged ≥1 month. Oral ondansetron is licensed from 6 months of age for the management of CINV, but the oral formulation is not recommended for PONV in children due to a lack of data.
- Ondansetron prolongs the QT interval in a dose-dependent manner. In addition, post-marketing cases of torsades de pointes have been reported in patients using ondansetron. Avoid ondansetron in patients with congenital long QT syndrome. Ondansetron should be administered with caution to patients who have or may develop prolongation of QTc, including patients with electrolyte abnormalities, congestive heart failure, or bradyarrhythmias, or patients taking other medicinal products that lead to QT prolongation or electrolyte abnormalities.
- Hypokalaemia and hypomagnesaemia should be corrected prior to ondansetron administration.

- Repeat iv doses of ondansetron should be given no less than 4h apart.
- Can cause constipation and headache.
- For iv infusion, dilute to a concentration of 320–640 micrograms/mL with 5% glucose or 0.9% NaCl or Ringer's solution; give over at least 15min.
- Available as: tablets (4mg, 8mg), oral lyophilisate (4mg, 8mg), oral syrup (4mg/5mL), and injection (2mg/mL, 2mL and 4mL ampoules).

Oxycodone

Uses
- Alternative opioid for severe pain.
- Pain of all types, unless opioid-insensitive.

Dose and routes
- Opioid switch: convert using OME from the previous opioid.
- Use the following *starting* doses in the opioid-naïve patient. The maximum dose stated applies to the *starting* dose only.

By mouth
Conversion
- po morphine 1.5:po oxycodone 1.
  - i.e. 15mg morphine:10mg oxycodone.
- *Child 1–12 months*: initial dose 50–125 micrograms/kg every 4–6h.
- *Child 1–12 years*: initial dose 125–200 micrograms/kg (maximum single dose 5mg) every 4–6h.
- *Child 12–18 years*: starting dose 5mg every 4–6h.
- Titrate as for morphine: increase the dose, if necessary, according to severity of pain.
- *Modified-release tablets, child 8–12 years*: initial dose 5mg every 12h, increased if necessary.
- *Modified-release tablets, child 12–18 years*: initial dose 10mg every 12h, increased if necessary.

By intravenous injection, subcutaneous injection, or continuous subcutaneous infusion
Conversion
- po to iv or sc oxycodone single bolus dose injection: divide the po oxycodone dose by 1.5.
- po to CSCI of oxycodone over 24h: divide the total daily dose of po oxycodone by 1.5.
- sc/iv morphine to sc/iv oxycodone ratio is ~1:1, i.e. use the same dose.
- Reason behind odd conversion ratio is bioavailability and rounding factors for safety.

Notes
- Opioid analgesic.
- Not licensed for use in children.

- It is important to prescribe breakthrough analgesia which is 5–10% of the total 24h dose given every 1–4h.
- It is moderately different from morphine in its structure, making it a candidate for opioid substitution.
- Caution in hepatic or renal impairment.
- Oxycodone injection may be given iv or sc as a bolus or by infusion. For CSCI, dilute with WFI, 0.9% NaCl, or 5% glucose.
- Oxycodone liquid may be administered via an enteral feeding tube.
- Schedule 2 CD.
- Available as: tablets and capsules (5mg, 10mg, 20mg), liquid (5mg/5mL, 10mg/mL), modified-release tablets (5mg, 10mg, 15mg, 20mg, 30mg, 40mg, 80mg, 120mg), and injection (10mg/mL and 50mg/mL).

Oxygen

Uses
- Breathlessness caused by hypoxaemia.
- Palliative care for symptom relief, including recognition of potential placebo effect.

Dose and routes
By inhalation through nasal cannula
- Flow rates of 1–2.5L/min, adjusted according to response. This will deliver between 24% and 35% oxygen, depending on the patient's breathing pattern and other factors. Lower flow rates may be appropriate, particularly for preterm neonates.

By inhalation through face mask
- Percentage inhaled oxygen is determined by the oxygen flow rate and/ or type of mask; 28% oxygen is usually recommended for continuous oxygen delivery.

Notes
- Oxygen saturations do not necessarily correlate with the severity of breathlessness. Where self-report is not possible, observation of the work of breathing is a more reliable indicator of breathlessness.
- Frequent or continuous measurement of oxygen saturations may lead to an over-reliance on technical data and distract from evaluation of the child's overall comfort, symptom relief, and well-being.
- Target oxygen saturations of 92–96% may be appropriate in acute illness but are not necessarily appropriate for palliative care. More usual target oxygen saturations are above 92% in long-term oxygen therapy, and 88–92% in children at risk of hypercapnic respiratory failure. Lower saturation levels may be tolerated in children with cyanotic congenital heart disease.
- It is important to be clear about the overall aims of oxygen treatment and realistic saturation levels for an individual child, as this will affect decisions about target oxygenation.

- In cyanotic congenital heart disease, oxygen has little effect in raising SaO_2 and is not generally indicated, although the degree of polycythaemia may be reduced. Pulmonary hypertension, in the early stages, may respond to oxygen, so it may be appropriate in the palliative care setting.
- Moving air, e.g. from a fan, may be equally effective in reducing the sensation of breathlessness when the child is not hypoxaemic.
- Nasal cannulae are generally preferable, as they allow the child to talk and eat with minimum restrictions. However, continuous nasal oxygen can cause drying of the nasal mucosa and dermatitis.
- Oxygen administration via a mask can be claustrophobic.
- The duration of supply from an oxygen cylinder will depend on the size of the cylinder and flow rate.
- An oxygen concentrator is recommended for patients requiring >8h of oxygen therapy per day.
- Liquid oxygen is more expensive but provides a longer duration of portable oxygen supply. Portable oxygen concentrators are now also available.
- If necessary, two concentrators can be Y-connected to supply very high oxygen concentrations.
- Higher concentrations of oxygen are required during air travel.
- Home oxygen order forms (HOOFs) and further information available from <mouse symbol> www.bprs.co.uk/oxygen.html.
- A secondary supply of oxygen for children spending a prolonged time away from home requires a second HOOF, available from the above website, e.g. short breaks, holiday, or extended periods with other relatives.

Pamidronate (disodium)

Uses
- Adjuvant analgesic for bone pain caused by metastatic disease.
- Adjuvant analgesic for bone pain in neurological and neuromuscular disorders, particularly due to osteopenia or osteoporosis.
- Tumour-induced hypercalcaemia.
- Treatment of secondary osteoporosis to reduce fracture risk.

NB. Evidence base is poor, but growing, for these uses in children. Seek specialist advice before use.

Dose and routes
- For bone pain (metastatic bone disease or osteopenia) and secondary osteoporosis, an effect on pain should be seen within 2 weeks but may need a year before definitive assessment. Continue dosing for as long as effective and tolerated or until substantial decline in performance status.

By intravenous infusion
- 1mg/kg as a single dose, infused over 4–6h, and repeated monthly as required; concentration not exceeding 60mg in 250mL, OR

- 1mg/kg infused over 4–6h on 3 consecutive days and repeated every 3 months as required; concentration not exceeding 60mg in 250mL.

For malignant hypercalcaemia (seek specialist advice)
By intravenous infusion
- 1mg/kg infused over 6h; concentration not exceeding 60mg in 250mL. Then repeated, as indicated, by corrected serum calcium.

Notes

- Not licensed for use in children. Well tolerated by children, but long-term effects unknown.
- Bisphosphonates have been used for some years in adults with bone metastases. It is becoming clear that they have a role in the wider causes of bone pain seen in children, particularly with neurological conditions.
- Current guidelines suggest an initial dose be given as an inpatient. Subsequent doses could be given at home, if the necessary medical and nursing support is available. May have worsening of pain at first.
- iv zoledronic acid can also be used.
- po risedronate and po alendronate—limited use for these indications, due to poor and variable bioavailability.
- If the iv route is unavailable, bisphosphonates can be administered by CSCI over 12–24h, together with sc hydration.
- Many bisphosphonates are available in different formulations, including oral, although absorption tends to be poor by the oral route and further reduced by food or fluids other than plain water.
- Caution: monitor renal function and electrolytes; ensure adequate hydration.
- Prolonged hypocalcaemia and hypomagnesaemia may occur with concurrent use of an aminoglycoside and a bisphosphonate. Consider calcium and vitamin D oral supplements to minimize potential risk of hypocalcaemia for those with mainly lytic bone metastases and at risk of calcium or vitamin D deficiency (e.g. through malabsorption or lack of exposure to sunlight).
- Risk of renal impairment is increased by concurrent use with other nephrotoxic drugs.
- Risk of atypical femoral fractures and of osteonecrosis, especially of jaw if pre-existing pathology. Recommend dental check pre-administration.
- Anecdotal risk of iatrogenic osteopetrosis with prolonged use (if prolonged use is likely, precede with dual-energy X-ray absorptiometry (DEXA) scan and investigation of calcium metabolism).
- Available as: injection vials for infusion of various volumes, at 3mg/mL, 6mg/mL, 9mg/mL, and 15mg/mL.

Paracetamol

Uses
- Mild to moderate pain.
- Pyrexia.

Dose and routes
The recommended indications and doses of paracetamol have been revised to take account of MHRA and Toxbase advice that paracetamol toxicity may occur with doses between 75mg and 150mg/kg/day (ingestion of over 150mg/kg/day is regarded as a definite risk of toxicity).

By mouth
- *Neonate 28–32 weeks corrected gestational age*: 20mg/kg as a single dose, then 10–15mg/kg every 8–12h, as necessary (maximum 30mg/kg/day in divided doses).
- *Neonates over 32 weeks corrected gestational age*: 20mg/kg as a single dose, then 10–15mg/kg every 6–8h, as necessary (maximum 60mg/kg/day in divided doses).
- *Child 1 month–6 years*: 20–30mg/kg as a single dose, then 15–20mg/kg every 4–6h, as necessary (maximum 75mg/kg/day in divided doses).
- *Child 6–12 years*: 20–30mg/kg (max 1g) as a single dose, then 15–20mg/kg every 4–6h, as necessary (maximum 75mg/kg/day or 4g/day in divided doses).
- *Over 12 years*: 15–20mg/kg (maximum 500mg to 1g) every 4–6h, as necessary (maximum 4g/day in divided doses).

Rectal
- *Neonate 28–32 weeks corrected gestational age*: 20mg/kg as a single dose, then 10–15mg/kg every 12h, as necessary (maximum 30mg/kg/day in divided doses).
- *Neonates over 32 weeks corrected gestational age*: 30mg/kg as a single dose, then 15–20mg/kg every 8h, as necessary (maximum 60mg/kg/day in divided doses).
- *Child 1–3 months*: 30mg/kg as a single dose, then 15–20mg/kg every 4–6h, as necessary (maximum 75mg/kg/day in divided doses).
- *Child 3 months to 12 years*: 30mg/kg as a single dose (maximum 1g), then 15–20mg/kg every 4–6h, as necessary (maximum 75mg/kg/day or 4g/day in divided doses).
- *Over 12 years*: 15–20mg/kg (maximum 500mg to 1g) every 4–6h, as necessary (maximum 4g/day in divided doses).

Intravenous: as infusion over 15min
- *Preterm neonate over 32 weeks corrected gestational age*: 7.5mg/kg every 8h, maximum 25mg/kg/day.
- *Neonate*: 10mg/kg every 4–6h (maximum 30mg/kg/day).
- *Infant and child body weight <10kg*: 10mg/kg every 4–6h (maximum 30mg/kg/day).

- *Child body weight 10–50kg*: 15mg/kg every 4–6h (maximum 60mg/kg/day).
- *Body weight over 50kg*: 1g every 4–6h (maximum 4g/day).

Notes

- Not licensed for use in children under 2 months by mouth; not licensed for use in preterm neonates by iv infusion; not licensed for use in children under 3 months by rectum; doses for severe symptoms not licensed; paracetamol oral suspension 500mg/5mL not licensed for use in children under 16 years.
- Oral and licensed rectal preparations are licensed for use in infants from 2 months for post-immunization pyrexia (single dose of 60mg which may be repeated once after 4–6h, if necessary) and from 3 months as antipyretic and analgesic.
- iv paracetamol is licensed for short-term treatment of moderate pain and of fever when other routes not possible.
- Consider use of non-pharmacological measures to relieve pain, as an alternative or in addition to analgesics.
- Hepatotoxic in overdose or prolonged high doses.
- In moderate renal impairment, use the maximum frequency of 6-hourly; in severe renal impairment, maximum frequency of 8-hourly.
- Many children and young people with life-limiting illness have low weight for their age. The doses above are therefore quoted mainly by weight, rather than by age (unlike most of the entries in the *BNF* and *BNFC*), in order to minimize the risk of overdosing in this patient group.
- Onset of action 15–30min po, 5–10min iv (analgesia), 30min iv (antipyretic). Duration of action 4–6h po and iv. Oral bioavailability 60–90%. Rectal bioavailability about two-thirds of oral. However, rectal absorption is now known to be erratic and incomplete, and results in slower absorption than oral administration (except in babies when the oral preparation used rectally speeds absorption, compared with suppositories). Elimination is slower in babies under 3 months.
- Dispersible tablets have high sodium content (over 14mmol per tablet), so caution with regular dosing (consider using the liquid preparation instead).
- For administration via an enteral feeding tube: use tablets dispersed in water for intragastric or intrajejunal administration. If the sodium content is problematic, use the liquid formulation. This can be used undiluted for intragastric administration; however, the viscosity of the paediatric liquid preparations is very high; it is difficult to administer these suspensions via a fine-bore tube without dilution. If administering intrajejunally, dilute with at least an equal quantity of water to reduce osmolarity and viscosity.
- For management of feverish illness in children, see updated NICE clinical guideline CG160. (Consider using *either* paracetamol or ibuprofen in children with fever who appear *distressed*, and consider changing to the other agent if distress is not alleviated. But do not use antipyretic agents with the sole aim of reducing the body temperature.) However, a recent Cochrane systematic review states 'there is some evidence that both alternating and combined antipyretic therapy may be more effective

at reducing temperatures than monotherapy alone'. For babies over 3 months, ibuprofen may be preferable to paracetamol, since asthma seems commoner in children who experienced early paracetamol exposure.
• Available as: tablets and caplets (500mg), capsules (500mg), soluble tablets (120mg, 500mg), oral suspension (120mg/5mL, 250mg/5mL), suppositories (60mg, 125mg, 250mg, 500mg, and other strengths available from 'specials' manufacturers or specialist importing companies), and iv infusion (10mg/mL in 50mL and 100mL vials).

Paraldehyde

Uses
• Treatment of prolonged seizures and status epilepticus.

Dose and routes
By rectal administration (dose shown is for premixed enema 50:50 with olive oil).
• *Neonate*: 0.8mL/kg as a single dose.
• *1 month to 18 years*: 0.8mL/kg (maximum 20mL) as a single dose.

Notes
• Rectal administration may cause irritation.
• Contraindicated in gastric disorders and colitis.
• Paraldehyde enema for rectal use is an unlicensed formulation and route of administration.
• Available as: paraldehyde enema—premixed solution of paraldehyde in olive oil in equal volumes from 'special-order' manufacturers or specialist importing companies.

Phenobarbital

Uses
• Adjuvant in pain of cerebral irritation.
• Control of terminal seizures.
• Sedation.
• Epilepsy, including status epilepticus. Commonly used first-line for seizures in neonates (phenytoin or benzodiazepine are the main alternatives).
• Agitation refractory to midazolam in end-of-life care.

Dose and routes
Status epilepticus/terminal seizures/agitation

Loading dose
• po, iv, or sc injection:
    • all ages: 20mg/kg/dose (maximum 1g) administered over 20min if by iv or sc injection (but see ➋ Notes below).

Subcutaneous or intravenous injection or infusion
- *Neonates for control of ongoing seizures*: 2.5–5mg/kg od or bd as maintenance.
- *Child 1 month to 12 years*: 2.5–5mg/kg (maximum single dose 300mg) od or bd or may be given as a continuous infusion over 24h.
- *Child 12–18 years*: 300mg bd or may be given as a continuous infusion over 24h.

Epilepsy
By mouth
- *Neonates for control of ongoing seizures*: 2.5–5mg/kg od or bd as maintenance.
- *Child 1 month to 12 years*: 1–1.5mg/kg bd, increased by 2mg/kg daily, as required (usual maintenance dose 2.5–4mg/kg od or bd).
- *Child 12–18 years*: 60–180mg od.

Notes
- Not licensed for agitation in end-of-life care.
- Single loading dose is required for initiation of therapy; administer via the enteral route, if possible. Loading dose can be administered iv over 20min or as a slow sc loading dose; however, the volume of the resultant solution will limit the rate at which an sc bolus can be administered.
- Loading dose essential to reach steady state quickly and avoid late toxicity due to accumulation.
- For patients already on po phenobarbital but needing parenteral treatment, doses equivalent to the patient's usual total daily dose of po phenobarbital can be used.
- Elimination half-life of 2–6 days in adults, 1–3 days in children.
- Phenobarbital induces various enzymes of the CYP450 system and thus may reduce the plasma concentrations of concomitant drugs that are metabolized by this system.
- Tablets may be crushed for administration, if preferred.
- Use a separate site to commence sc infusion. sc bolus injections should be avoided, because they can cause tissue necrosis due to the high pH.
- It is essential to dilute the injection in ten times the volume of water for injection before iv or sc injection (i.e. to the concentration of 20mg/mL).
- Available as: tablets (15mg, 30mg, 60mg), oral elixir (15mg/5mL), and injection (15mg/mL, 60mg/mL, and 200mg/mL). The licensed oral elixir of 15mg in 5mL contains alcohol 38%, and it is preferable to obtain an alcohol-free oral liquid via one of the specials manufacturers.

Phenytoin

Uses
- Epilepsy (third- or fourth-line oral anti-epileptic), including for status epilepticus.
- Neuropathic pain (effective, at least short-term, but not used first-line).

Dose and routes
All forms of epilepsy (including tonic–clonic, focal, and neonatal seizures), except absence seizures; neuropathic pain.

Oral or slow intravenous injection
- *Neonate*: initial loading dose by slow iv injection 18mg/kg, THEN by mouth 2.5–5mg/kg bd, adjusted according to response and plasma phenytoin levels. Usual maximum 7.5mg/kg bd.
- *Child 1 month to 12 years*: initial dose of 1.5–2.5mg/kg bd, then adjust according to response and plasma phenytoin levels to 2.5–5mg/kg bd as a usual target maintenance dose. Usual maximum dose of 7.5mg/kg bd or 300mg daily.
- *Child 12–18 years*: initial dose of 75–150mg bd, then adjusted according to response and plasma phenytoin levels to 150–200mg bd as a usual target maintenance dose. Usual maximum dose of 300mg bd.

Status epilepticus and acute symptomatic seizures
Slow intravenous injection or infusion
- *Neonate*: 20mg/kg loading dose over at least 20min, then 2mg/kg/dose (over 30min) every 8–12h as a usual maintenance dose in the first week of life. Adjust according to response, and older babies may need higher doses. After the first dose, po doses usually as effective as iv in babies over 2 weeks old.
- *Child 1 month to 12 years*: 20mg/kg loading dose over at least 20min, then 2.5–5mg/kg bd usual maintenance dose.
- *Child 12–18 years*: 20mg/kg loading dose over at least 20min, then up to 100mg (over 30min) 3–4 times daily usual maintenance dose.

Notes
- Licensed status: suspension 90mg in 5mL is a 'special' and unlicensed. Other preparations are licensed for use in children as an anticonvulsant (age range not specified).
- Phenytoin acts as a membrane stabilizer.
- It has a narrow therapeutic index and an unpredictable half-life, and the relationship between the dose and plasma drug concentration is non-linear. The rate of elimination is also very variable, especially in the first few weeks and months of life. Co-treatment with commonly used drugs can significantly alter the half-life.

- Phenytoin has numerous interactions with other drugs due to hepatic enzyme induction. Long-term use is associated with significant side effects. It is no more effective than other anti-epileptics and hence not usually used first-line, although it does enable rapid titration.
- Continuous ECG and BP monitoring required during iv administration.
- Oral bioavailability of 90–95% is roughly equivalent to iv, plasma half-life 7–42h. Poor rectal absorption.
- Absorption is exceptionally poor via the jejunal route.
- Reduce dose in hepatic impairment. Monitor carefully if reduced albumin or protein binding, e.g. in renal failure.
- Caution: cross-sensitivity is reported with carbamazepine.
- Avoid abrupt withdrawal.
- Consider vitamin D supplementation in patients who are immobilized for long periods or who have inadequate sun exposure or dietary intake of calcium.
- Before and after administration, flush iv line with 0.9% NaCl.
- For *iv injection*, give into a large vein at a rate not exceeding 1mg/kg/min (maximum 50mg/min).
- For *iv infusion*, dilute to a concentration not exceeding 10mg/mL with 0.9% NaCl, and give into a large vein through an in-line filter (0.22–0.50 micrometres) at a rate not exceeding 1mg/kg/min (maximum 50mg/min); complete administration within 1h of preparation.
- Prescriptions for oral preparations should include the brand name and be of consistent preparation type, to ensure consistency of drug delivery.
- Preparations containing phenytoin sodium are *not* bioequivalent to those containing phenytoin base (such as Epanutin Infatabs® and Epanutin® suspension); 100mg of phenytoin sodium is approximately equivalent in therapeutic effect to 92mg phenytoin base. The dose is the same for all phenytoin products when initiating therapy; however, if switching between these products, the difference in phenytoin content may be clinically significant. Care is needed when making changes between formulations, and plasma phenytoin concentration monitoring is recommended.
- Bioavailability may be reduced unpredictably by enteral feeds and/or NG tube feeds, so flush with water to enhance absorption; interrupt enteral feeding for at least 1–2h before and after giving phenytoin, and maintain similar timings and regimes from day to day.
- Available as: tablets (phenytoin sodium 100mg, generic), capsules (Epanutin® phenytoin sodium 25mg, 50mg,100mg, 300mg), Epanutin Infatabs® (chewable tablets of phenytoin base 50mg), oral suspension (Epanutin® phenytoin base 30mg/5mL, and 90mg/5mL phenytoin base available as an 'unlicensed special'), and injection (phenytoin sodium 50mg/mL, generic).

Phosphate (rectal enema)

Uses
- Constipation refractory to other treatments.

Dose and routes
By rectal enema
- *Child 3–7 years*: 45–65mL od.
- *Child 7–12 years*: 65–100mL od.
- *Child 12–18 years*: 100–128mL od.

Notes
- Maintain good hydration, and watch for electrolyte imbalance.
- Contraindicated in acute gastrointestinal conditions (including gastrointestinal obstruction, inflammatory bowel disease, and conditions associated with increased colonic absorption).
- Use only after specialist advice.
- Available as Phosphate enema BP formula B in 128mL with a standard or long rectal tube (NB. alternative Fleet® Ready-to-use Enema requires slightly different dosing: 40–60mL for ages 3–7y, 60–90mL for ages 7–12y, and 90–118mL for ages 12–18y).

Promethazine

Uses
- Sleep disturbance.
- Mild sedation.
- Antihistamine.
- Can also be used to treat nausea and vomiting, and vertigo.

Dose and routes (for promethazine hydrochloride)
By mouth

Symptomatic relief of allergy
- *Child 2–5 years*: 5mg bd or 5–15mg at night.
- *Child 5–10 years*: 5–10mg bd or 10–25mg at night.
- *Child 10–18 years*: 10–20mg 2–3 times daily or 25mg at night, increased to 25mg bd, if necessary.

Sedation (short-term use)
- *Child 2–5 years*: 15–20mg at night.
- *Child 5–10 years*: 20–25mg at night.
- *Child 10–18 years*: 25–50mg at night.

Nausea and vomiting (particularly in anticipation of motion sickness)
- *Child 2–5 years*: 5mg bd.
- *Child 5–10 years*: 10mg bd.
- *Child 10–18 years*: 20–25mg bd.

Notes

- Antimuscarinic phenothiazine antihistamine, also with D_2 antagonist activity.
- Not for use in under 2 years due to risk of fatal respiratory depression.
- Note drug interactions, particularly causing increased antimuscarinic and sedative effects.
- Caution in epilepsy.
- Can be effective for up to 12h. Drowsiness may wear off after a few days of treatment.
- For use by feeding tube: the elixir is slightly viscous so can be mixed with an equal volume of water to reduce viscosity and resistance to flushing. Tablets will disintegrate if shaken in water for 5min.
- Available as: promethazine hydrochloride tablets (10mg, 25mg), oral elixir (5mg/5mL), and injection (25mg/mL). (Promethazine teoclate tablets also available, 25mg, licensed for nausea, vomiting, and labyrinthine disorders. Dosing slightly different.)

Quinine sulfate

Uses

- Leg cramps.

Dose and routes

By mouth

- Not licensed or recommended for children, as no experience.
- *Adult dose*: quinine sulfate 200mg at bedtime, increased to 300mg if necessary.

Notes

- Not licensed for use in children for this condition.
- Moderate evidence indicates it to be more effective than placebo in reducing frequency and intensity of cramp.
- Regulatory agencies consider that, given that alternatives to quinine are available, the risks associated with its use are unacceptably high. Rare, but serious, side effects include thrombocytopenia and haemolytic uraemic syndrome. Also very toxic in overdose and has serious interactions with warfarin and digoxin. Therefore, MHRA advises that quinine should only be used if the four criteria are all met: treatable causes have been ruled out; non-pharmacological measures have failed; cramps regularly cause loss of sleep; and they are very painful or frequent. Patients should be monitored for signs of thrombocytopenia in the early stages of treatment.
- If used, treatment should be discontinued after 4 weeks if ineffective, and interrupted every 3 months to re-evaluate benefit.
- Available as: tablets (200mg quinine sulfate).

Ranitidine

Uses

- Gastro-oesophageal reflux.
- Treatment of gastritis, benign gastric, and duodenal ulcers.
- Gastro-protection (e.g. with combination NSAID/steroids).
- Other conditions requiring reduction in gastric acid.

Dose and routes

By mouth

- *Neonate*: 2–3mg/kg tds (absorption unreliable).
- *Child 1–6 months*: 1mg/kg tds, increasing, if necessary, to maximum 3mg/kg tds.
- *Child 6 months to 3 years*: 2–4mg/kg bd.
- *Child 3–12 years*: 2–4mg/kg (maximum single dose 150mg) bd. Dose may be increased up to 5mg/kg (maximum 300mg/dose) bd in severe GORD.
- *Child 12–18 years*: 150mg bd or 300mg at night. May be increased, if necessary, in moderate to severe GORD to 300mg bd or 150mg qds for up to 12 weeks.

By slow iv injection, diluted to 2.5mg/mL, and given over at least 3min (some adult centres give as sc injection—unlicensed route):
- *neonate*: 0.5–1mg/kg every 6–8h (may need 2mg/kg 8-hourly, as variable first-pass metabolism affects uptake);
- *child 1 month to 18 years*: 1mg/kg (maximum 50mg) every 6–8h (may be given as an intermittent infusion at a rate of 25mg/h).

Notes

- Oral formulations not licensed for use in children <3 years; injection not licensed for children under 6 months.
- Use gastric pH to judge best dose in early infancy.
- PPIs, H2 antagonists, and prokinetics all relieve symptoms of non-ulcer dyspepsia and acid reflux, PPIs being the most effective. PPIs and 'double-dose' H2 antagonists are effective at preventing NSAID-related endoscopic peptic ulcers. Adding a bedtime dose of H2 antagonist to a high-dose PPI may improve nocturnal acid reflux, but evidence is poor.
- Time to peak plasma concentration is 2–3h, half-life 2–3h, duration of action 8–12h.
- Ranitidine may increase the plasma concentration of midazolam.
- May cause rebound hyperacidity at night.
- Via feeding tubes, use effervescent tablets as first choice, unless sodium content is a concern. Use oral liquid as alternative. (Standard tablets do not disperse readily in water.)
- Can use iv, if needed, in severe nausea and vomiting. Some centres use sc doses bd to qds.
- Available as: tablets and effervescent tablets (150mg, 300mg), oral solution (75mg/5mL), and injection (25mg/mL).

Risperidone

Uses

- Dystonia and dystonic spasms refractory to first- and second-line treatment.
- Psychotic tendency/crises in Batten's disease.
- Has antiemetic activity (some experience in refractory nausea and vomiting in adults; not evaluated in children).
- Treatment of mania or psychosis under specialist supervision.

Dose and routes

Oral

- *Child 5–12 years (weight 20–50kg)*: 250 micrograms od; increasing, if necessary, in steps of 250 micrograms on alternate days to a maximum of 750 micrograms daily.
- *Child 12 years or over (>50kg)*: 500 micrograms od; increasing in steps of 500 micrograms on alternate days to a maximum of 1.5mg daily.
  - In juvenile Batten's disease, may need 500 micrograms daily, increasing to 1.5mg tds during crises with hallucinations—this dose can be reduced or stopped, as symptoms settle (episodes usually last 1–6 weeks).

Notes

- Not licensed for use in children for these indications. Risperidone is licensed for the short-term symptomatic treatment (up to 6 weeks) of persistent aggression in conduct disorder in children from the age of 5 years.
- 99% bioavailable; 1–2h to peak plasma concentration. Onset of action hours to days in delirium; days to weeks in psychosis. Plasma half-life 24h. Duration of action 12–48h.
- Caution in epilepsy and cardiovascular disease; extrapyramidal symptoms less frequent than with older antipsychotic medications; withdraw gradually after prolonged use. Risperidone can cause significant weight gain.
- Initial and subsequent doses should be halved in renal or hepatic impairment.
- Tablets disintegrate in water within 5min for easy administration via enteral feeding tubes. The oral liquid is simple to administer via a feeding tube.
- Available as: tablets (500 micrograms, 1mg, 2mg, 3mg, 4mg, 6mg), orodispersible tablets (500 micrograms, 1mg, 2mg, 3mg, 4mg), and liquid (1mg/mL).

Salbutamol

Uses
- Wheezing/breathlessness caused by bronchospasm.
- Also used in hyperkalaemia, for prevention and treatment of chronic lung disease in premature infants, and sometimes in muscular disorders or muscle weakness (seek specialist advice, not covered here).

Dose and routes
For exacerbation of reversible airway obstruction and prevention of allergen- or exercise-induced bronchospasm
(NB. See separate detailed guidance in standard texts for use in acute asthma.)

Aerosol inhalation
- *Child 1 month to 18 years*: 100–200 micrograms (1–2 puffs) for persistent symptoms up to qds.

Nebulized solution
- *Neonate*: 1.25–2.5mg up to qds.
- *Child 1 month to 18 years*: 2.5–5mg up to qds.

Oral preparations (but use by inhalation preferred for treatment of bronchospasm)
- *Child 1 month to 2 years*: 100 micrograms/kg (maximum 2mg) 3–4 times daily.
- *Child 2–6 years*: 1–2mg 3–4 times daily.
- *Child 6–12 years*: 2mg 3–4 times daily.
- *Child 12–18 years*: 2–4mg 3–4 times daily.

Notes
- Salbutamol is not licensed for use in hyperkalaemia; syrup and tablets are not licensed for use in children <2 years; modified-release tablets are not licensed for use in children <3 years; injection is not licensed for use in children.
- In palliative care, if airflow obstruction is suspected, a pragmatic approach may be to give a trial (e.g. 1–2 weeks) of a bronchodilator and evaluate the impact on symptoms. Spirometry should normally be used to confirm a possible underlying asthma diagnosis.
- Salbutamol has not been shown to be effective in children <2 years, presumably due to the immaturity of the receptors; ipratropium may be more helpful in those <1–2 years.
- For an acute episode, many paediatricians now advise multi-dosing of salbutamol 100 micrograms up to ten times, via a spacer where practicable for the patient, instead of a nebulizer.
- Side effects: increased heart rate; feeling 'edgy' or agitated; tremor.
- The side effects listed above may prevent use, in which case ipratropium bromide is a good alternative.

- Inhaled product should be used with a suitable spacer device, and the child/carer should be given appropriate training. Inhaler technique should be explained and checked. The HFA (hydrofluoroalkane) propellant now used in multi-dose inhalers tends to clog the nozzle, so weekly cleaning is recommended.
- Salbutamol nebules are intended to be used undiluted. However, if prolonged delivery time (>10min) is required, the solution may be diluted with sterile 0.9% NaCl. Salbutamol can be mixed with a nebulized solution of ipratropium bromide.
- Available as: nebulizer solution (2.5mg in 2.5mL, 5mg in 2.5mL), respirator solution (5mg in 1mL), and aerosol inhalation (100 micrograms/puff) by metered dose inhaler (MDI), with various spacer devices. Various types of dry powder inhaler are also available. Also available as salbutamol tablets (costly) 2mg and 4mg, modified-release capsules 4mg and 8mg, and oral solution 2mg/5mL. Preparations for injection (500 micrograms/mL) and iv infusion (1mg/mL) are also available.

Senna

Uses
- Constipation.

Dose and routes
By mouth
Initial doses which can be adjusted according to response and tolerance.
- *Child 1 month to 2 years*: 0.5mL/kg (maximum 2.5mL) of syrup od.
- *Child 2–6 years*: 2.5–5mL of syrup a day.
- *Child 6–12 years*: 5–10mL a day of syrup or 1–2 tablets at night or 2.5–5mL of granules.
- *Child 12–18 years*: 10–20mL a day of syrup or 2–4 tablets at night or 5–10mL of granules.

Notes
- Syrup is not licensed for use in children <2 years, and tablets/granules are not licensed for use in children <6 years.
- Stimulant laxative.
- Onset of action 8–12h.
- Initial dose should be low, then increased, if necessary.
- Doses can be exceeded on specialist advice.
- Granules can be mixed in hot milk or sprinkled on food.
- Oral liquid may be administered via an enteral feeding tube.
- Available as: tablets (7.5mg sennoside B), oral syrup (7.5mg/5mL sennoside B), and granules (15mg/5mL sennoside B).

Sodium citrate

Uses
- Constipation where osmotic laxative indicated.

Dose and routes
Micolette Micro-enema®
Enema, sodium citrate 450mg, sodium lauryl sulfoacetate 45mg, glycerol 625mg, together with citric acid, potassium sorbate, and sorbitol in a viscous solution, in 5mL.
- *By rectum, child 3–18 years*: 5–10mL as a single dose.

Micralax Micro-enema®
Enema, sodium citrate 450mg, sodium alkylsulfoacetate 45mg, sorbic acid 5mg, together with glycerol and sorbitol in a viscous solution, in 5mL.
- *By rectum, child 3–18 years*: 5mL as a single dose.

Relaxit Micro-enema®
Enema, sodium citrate 450mg, sodium lauryl sulfate 75mg, sorbic acid 5mg, together with glycerol and sorbitol in a viscous solution, in a 5mL single-dose pack with nozzle.
- *By rectum: child 1 month to 18 years*: 5mL as a single dose (insert only half nozzle length in a child under 3 years).

Notes
- For under 3 years, insert only half nozzle length.
- Available as: micro-enema (5mL).

Sodium picosulfate

Uses
- Constipation.

Dose and routes
By mouth
- *Child 1 month–4 years*: initial dose of 2.5mg od, increasing, if necessary, according to response to a suggested maximum of 10mg daily.
- *Child 4–18 years*: initial dose of 2.5mg od, increasing, if necessary, according to response to a suggested maximum of 20mg daily.

Notes
- Elixir is licensed for use in children of all ages; capsules are not licensed for use in children <4 years of age.
- Acts as a stimulant laxative.
- Onset of action 6–12h.
- Effectiveness dependent upon breakdown by gut flora—previous effectiveness may therefore be lost during courses of antibiotics and ensuing altered gut flora.

- For administration via an enteral feeding tube: use the liquid preparation; dilute with an equal volume of water prior to administration. Sodium picosulfate reaches the colon without any significant absorption; therefore, the therapeutic response will be unaffected by jejunal administration.
- Available as: elixir (5mg/5mL) and capsules (2.5mg).

Sucralfate

Uses
- Stress ulcer prophylaxis.
- Prophylaxis against bleeding from oesophageal or gastric varices; adjunct in the treatment of: oesophagitis with evidence of mucosal ulceration, gastric or duodenal ulceration, upper gastrointestinal bleeding of unknown cause.

Dose and routes
Oral

Stress ulcer prophylaxis, prophylaxis against bleeding from oesophageal or gastric varices
- *Child 1 month to 2 years*: 250mg 4–6 times daily.
- *Child 2–12 years*: 500mg 4–6 times daily.
- *Child 12–15 years*: 1g 4–6 times daily.
- *Child 15–18 years*: 1g six times daily (maximum 8g/day).

Oesophagitis with evidence of mucosal ulceration, or gastric or duodenal ulceration
- *Child 1 month to 2 years*: 250mg 4–6 times daily.
- *Child 2–12 years*: 500mg 4–6 times daily.
- *Child 12–15 years*: 1g 4–6 times daily.
- *Child 15–18 years*: 2g bd (on rising and at bedtime) or 1g qds (1h before meals and at bedtime) taken for 4–6 weeks (up to 12 weeks in resistant cases); maximum 8g daily.

Notes
- Not licensed for use in children <15 years; tablets are not licensed for prophylaxis of stress ulceration.
- Administer 1h before meals.
- Spread doses evenly throughout waking hours.
- *Bezoar formation*: following reports of bezoar formation associated with sucralfate, the CSM has advised caution in seriously ill patients, especially those receiving concomitant enteral feeds or those with predisposing conditions such as delayed gastric emptying.
- Caution—absorption of aluminium from sucralfate may be significant in patients on dialysis or with renal impairment.
- Tablets may be crushed and dispersed in water.

- Administration of sucralfate suspension and enteral feeds via an NG or gastrostomy tube should be separated by *at least* 1h. In rare cases, bezoar formation has been reported when sucralfate suspension and enteral feeds have been given too closely together.
- Caution—sucralfate oral suspension may block fine-bore feeding tubes.
- Available as: oral suspension (1g in 5mL) and tablets (1g).

Temazepam

Uses
- Sleep disturbance where anxiety is a cause.

Dose and routes
By mouth
- *Adult*: 10–20mg at night. Dose may be increased to 40mg at night in exceptional circumstances.

Notes
- Not licensed for use in children.
- Oral solution may be administered via an enteral feeding tube.
- Available as: tablets (10mg, 20mg) and oral solution (10mg/5mL).
- Schedule 3 CD.

Tizanidine

Uses
- Skeletal muscle relaxant.
- Chronic severe muscle spasm or spasticity.

Dose and routes
- *Child 18 months to 7 years*: 1mg/day; increase, if necessary, according to response.
- *Child 7–12 years*: 2mg/day; increase, if necessary, according to response.
- *Child >12 years*: as per adult dose—initially 2mg, increasing in increments of 2mg at intervals of 3–4 days. Give the total daily dose in divided doses up to 3–4 times daily. Usual total daily dose 24mg. Maximum total daily dose 36mg.

Notes
- Not licensed for use in children.
- Usually prescribed and titrated by neurologists.
- Timing and frequency of dosing are individual to the specific patient, as maximal effect is seen after 2–3h and is short-lived.
- Use with caution in liver disease; monitor liver function regularly.
- Use with caution with drugs known to prolong the QT interval.
- Avoid abrupt withdrawal—risk of rebound hypertension and tachycardia.

- Tizanidine plasma concentrations are increased by CYP1A2 inhibitors, potentially leading to severe hypotension.
- Drowsiness, weakness, and dry mouth are common side effects.
- Tablets may be crushed and administered in water, if preferred. May be administered via an enteral feeding tube. Tablets do not disperse readily but will disintegrate if shaken in 10mL of water for 5min. The resulting dispersion will flush via an 8Fr NG tube, without blockage.
- Available as: tablets (2mg, 4mg).

Tramadol

The WHO now advises there is insufficient evidence to make a recommendation for an alternative to codeine (tramadol) and recommends moving directly from non-opioids (step 1) to low-dose strong opioids for the management of moderate uncontrolled pain in children.

Uses
- Minor opioid with additional non-opioid analgesic actions.

Dose and routes
By mouth
- *Child 5–12 years*: 1–2mg/kg every 4–6h (maximum initial single dose of 50mg; maximum of four doses in 24h). Increase, if necessary, to a maximum dose of 3mg/kg (maximum single dose 100mg) every 6h.
- *Child 12–18 years*: initial dose of 50mg every 4–6h. Increase, if necessary, to a maximum of 400mg/day, given in divided doses every 4–6h.

By intravenous injection or infusion
- *Child 5–12 years*: 1–2mg/kg every 4–6h (maximum initial single dose of 50mg; maximum four doses in 24h). Increase, if necessary, to a maximum dose of 3mg/kg (maximum single dose 100mg) every 6h.
- *Child 12–18 years*: initial dose of 50mg every 4–6h. Dose may be increased, if necessary, to 100mg every 4–6h. Maximum 600mg/day in divided doses.

Notes
- Not licensed for use in children <12 years.
- Tramadol is a Schedule 3 CD, but exempted from safe custody requirements.
- By mouth, tramadol is about one-tenth as potent as morphine.
- Onset of action after an oral dose is 30–60min. Duration of action is 4–9h.
- Causes less constipation and respiratory depression than the equivalent morphine dose.
- Analgesic effect is reduced by ondansetron.

- Soluble or orodispersible tablets may be dissolved in water for administration via an enteral feeding tube.
- Available as: capsules (50mg, 100mg), soluble tablets (50mg), orodispersible tablets (50mg), modified-release tablets and capsules (100mg, 150mg, 200mg, 300mg, 400mg), oral drops (100mg/mL), and injection (50mg/mL).

Tranexamic acid

Uses
- Oozing of blood (e.g. from mucous membranes/capillaries), particularly when due to low or dysfunctional platelets.
- Menorrhagia.

Dose and routes
By mouth

Inhibition of fibrinolysis
- *Child 1 month to 18 years*: 15–25mg/kg (maximum 1.5 g) 2–3 times daily.

Menorrhagia
- *Child 12–18 years*: 1g tds for up to 4 days. If very heavy bleeding, a maximum daily dose of 4g (in divided doses) may be used. Treatment should not be initiated until menstruation has started.

By intravenous injection over at least 10min
Inhibition of fibrinolysis
- *Child 1 month to 18 years*: 10mg/kg (maximum 1g) 2–3 times a day.

By continuous intravenous infusion
Inhibition of fibrinolysis
- *Child 1 month to 18 years*: 45mg/kg over 24h.

Mouthwash 5% solution
- *Child 6–18 years*: 5–10mL qds for 2 days. Not to be swallowed.

Topical treatment
- Apply gauze soaked in 100mg/mL of injection solution to the affected area.

Notes
- Injection not licensed for use in children under 1 year or for administration by iv infusion.
- Can cause clot 'colic' if used in presence of haematuria.
- Parenteral preparation can be used topically.
- Available as: tablets (500mg), syrup (500mg/5mL available from 'specials' manufacturers), and injection (100mg/mL 5mL ampoules). Mouthwash only as extemporaneous preparation.

Trihexyphenidyl

Uses
- Dystonias; sialorrhoea (drooling); antispasmodic.

Dose and routes
Oral
- *Child 3 months to 18 years*: initial dose of 1–2mg daily in 1–2 divided doses, increased every 3–7 days by 1mg daily; adjusted according to response and side effects; maximum 2mg/kg/daily (maximum 70mg/daily).

Generally, the doses needed to control drooling are much lower than those needed for dystonias.

Notes
- Anticholinergic agent thought to act through partially blocking central (striatal) cholinergic receptors.
- Not licensed for use in children.
- Use in conjunction with careful observation and a full non-drug management programme, including positioning, massage, holding, distraction, checking for causes of exacerbations, etc. Advisable to seek specialist neurological input before use of trihexyphenidyl.
- Side effects are very common, and it is important to start at a low dose and increase gradually to minimize the incidence and severity. Mouth dryness, gastrointestinal disturbance, blurring of vision, dizziness, and nausea can occur in 30–50% patients. Less common side effects include urinary retention, tachycardia, and, with very high doses, CNS disturbance.
- Use with caution in children with renal or hepatic impairment.
- Onset of action is usually within 1h; maximum effect occurs within 2–3h, and duration of effect ~6–12h.
- May take several weeks for maximal effect on dystonic movements to be seen.
- Do not withdraw abruptly in children who have been on long-term treatment.
- Tablets may be crushed and mixed in soft food.
- For administration via a gastrostomy, the liquid may be used or the tablets will disperse readily in water.
- Available as: tablets (2mg and 5mg) and oral liquid (pink syrup; 5mg in 5mL).

Vitamin K (phytomenadione)

Uses
- Treatment of haemorrhage associated with vitamin K deficiency (seek specialist advice).

Dose and routes
By mouth or intravenous
- *Neonate*: 100 micrograms/kg.
- *Child 1 month to 18 years*: 250–300 micrograms/kg (maximum 10mg) as a single dose.

Notes
- Caution with iv use in premature infants <2.5kg.
- Available as Konakion® MM injection 10mg/mL (1mL ampoule) for slow iv injection or iv infusion in 5% glucose; NOT for im injection.
- Available as Konakion® MM Paediatric 10mg/mL (0.2mL ampoule) for po administration or im injection. Also for slow iv injection or iv infusion in 5% glucose.
- There is not a UK licensed formulation of vitamin K tablets currently available. Possible to obtain 10mg phytomenadione tablets via a specialist importation company.

Index